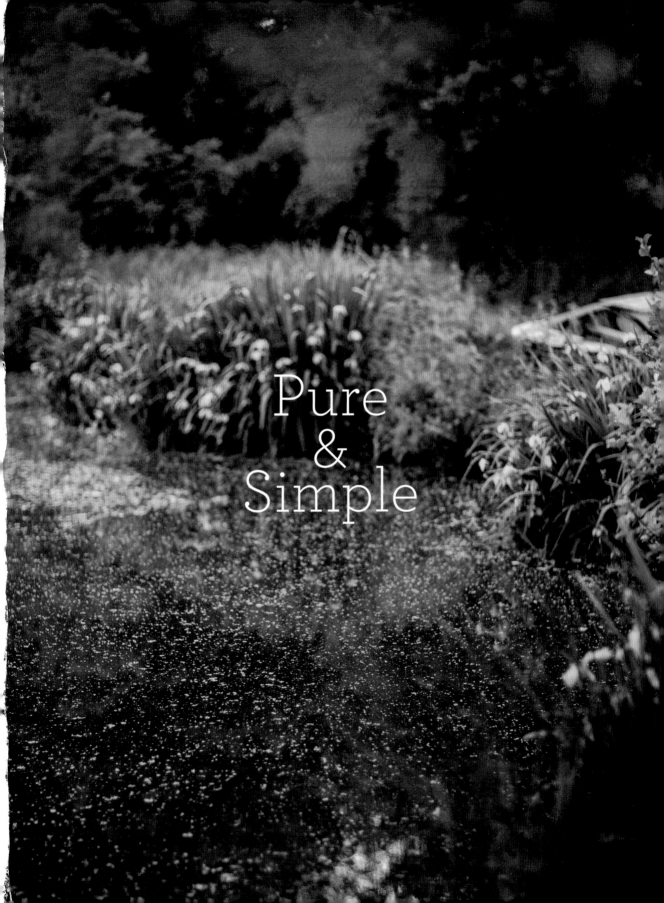

Pure
&
Simple

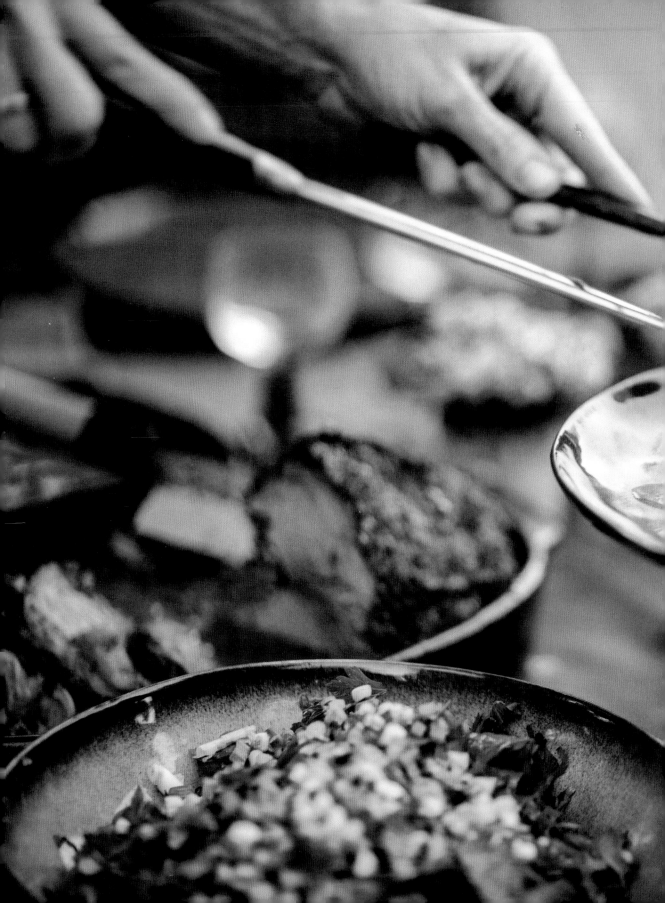

Pure
&
Simple

A NATURAL FOOD
WAY OF LIFE

PASCALE
NAESSENS

Abrams, New York

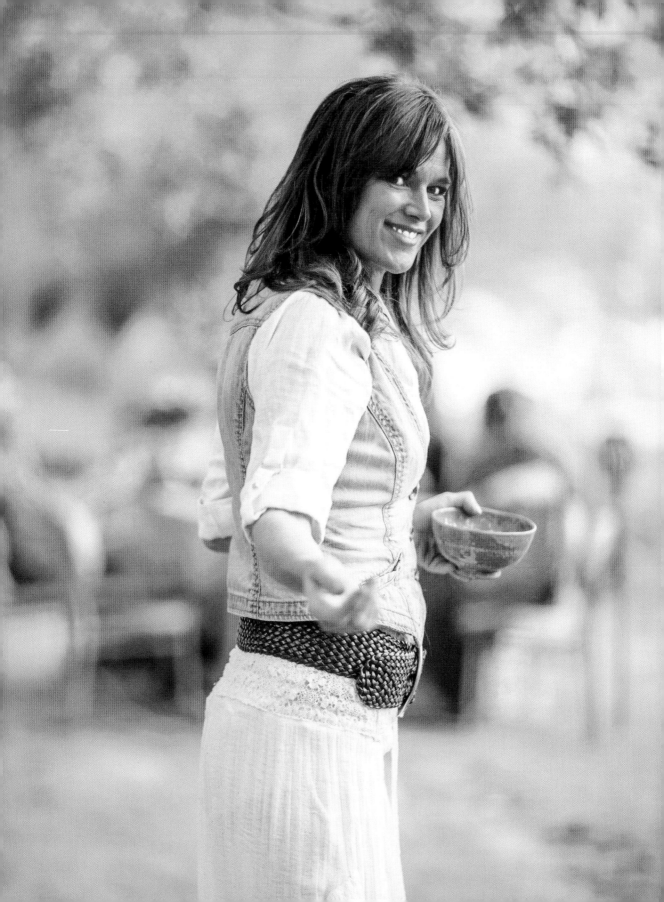

Contents

The Science of Eating Well

WE BEGAN TO BETTER UNDERSTAND WHY CERTAIN DISEASES OCCUR after we started to examine our evolutionary background. Evolutionary medicine is the science aimed at answering these questions. As famously explained by Charles Darwin, natural selection allowed for the genes of individuals who were best adapted (survival of the fittest) to the prehistoric conditions of existence to be encoded in our DNA.

Man is also genetically adapted to, and thus most healthy in, his natural, primal environment. In the ten thousand years since the agricultural revolution, and especially in the last hundred or so years since the Industrial Revolution and the development of fast food, we have made changes to our environment at a quicker pace than the human body can adapt. These rapid changes have disrupted the ancient balance between our genes and our environment. The resulting "mismatch" is the cause of many of our diseases, including obesity, cardiovascular diseases, and cancer.

To be able to maintain our health as we age, we must go back to our primal environment. However, what was this primal environment—what Darwin called our "conditions of existence"—that made us transition from ape to man? What distinguishes us from our closest relatives, the chimpanzees, is our enormously large and complex brain. When our early forefathers left the jungle and settled on fertile riverbanks and coastlines, the optimal conditions were created for the development of this highly advanced brain. Food from this land-water ecosystem contained various nutrients that were essential to this development.

In the following six million years, the human brain tripled in volume, and our genes adjusted gradually to living by the water. Then, man conquered the world by spreading across coastlines, lakes, rivers, creeks, and streams; the land-water ecosystem remained the main source of food, always and everywhere. Our primal environment is the land-water ecosystem, and the food that we find in and along the water is the food we need to eat to remain healthy into old age.

Pascale puts this scientific knowledge into practice. With her delicious recipes, she restores harmony between our primal genes and our modern environment, making us fit, energetic, and healthy. Moreover, she contributes her part to reducing the ever-rising cost of healthcare. By restoring balance between our genes and our food, the focus is less on treating than on preventing diseases. And this is what it's all about: If you are healthy, you are truly happy!

—Dr. Remko Kuipers

Remko Kuipers is a physician and a pharmacist. He has a doctorate in evolutionary medicine with a focus on our primal nutrition. He gives international lectures on his studies and is the author of *Het oerdieet* (*The Primal Diet*).

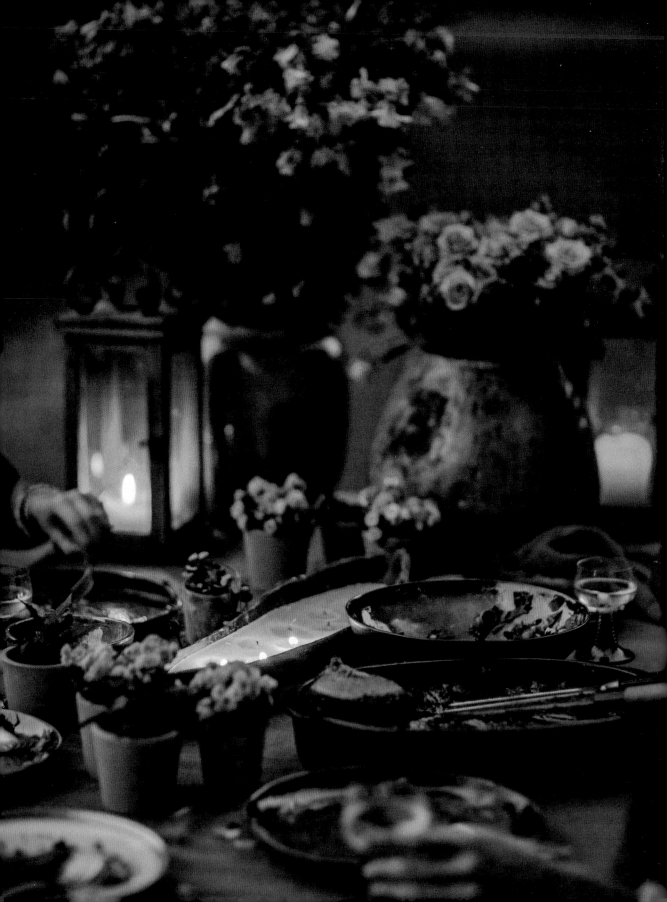

Food: A Source of Happiness

Many people may not believe me, but I once had an eating disorder—like so many models. "Eat fewer calories and exercise more." I heard this so often and tried many times to conform to this rule. I struggled with my eating habits for years. I was constantly hungry and never satisfied.

Fortunately, today, things are very different: I eat a lot more, I don't count calories, I feel wonderfully satisfied after each meal, and I love my healthy, lean body. Why are things working for me now, and not then? My willpower hasn't changed. What has changed is that I no longer listen to classic nutritional advice, but have adopted a new, up-to-date approach to eating that I will share with you in the following pages. As Professor Dariush Mozaffarian, the world-renowned nutritionist from Boston, said to me: "Nutrition is a science and science evolves. You don't want to take pills from ten years ago anymore, do you?"

Liberated from my eating disorder, for a few years I was euphoric. But when I saw people around me, and especially young girls suffering as I had done, my heart ached. That's when I started looking for a way to share my experience because I knew I would be able to help people who were in the same situation as I had been. If I was able to free myself from my carbohydrate addiction, then anyone could. That's when the idea came to me to write a cookbook about eating differently, using the latest nutritional insights.

Since then, I have published seven bestselling books in Belgium, selling more than one and a half million copies combined, and so many people have found their way to a healthier, more energetic, and "lighter" life through my books. My books have helped create a real culinary movement—people are once again free to enjoy their food, but still stay slim and healthy. I think my readers are also attracted to my romantic way of cooking, because the delicious and simple recipes are uncomplicated, easily accessible, and designed to share with friends and family. I'm thrilled to have the opportunity to have this book published in English, so that I can share my message with a new audience.

THIS BOOK IS NOT JUST ABOUT HEALTHY FOOD.

I want it all. I want to:
– share meals with friends,
– not spend too much time in the kitchen,
– and not put on weight.

I don't want to turn anything down. And this book is a reflection of my hunger to live a good life and an introduction to my way of getting all of the above.

The best moments in life often occur at the table. A romantic dinner, chatting with friends, catching up over a glass of wine—I wouldn't miss those moments for the world. And these experiences are actually the reason I enjoy cooking—bringing people together and enjoying time together. But I'm also always conscious of my own enjoyment: I don't want complicated recipes that keep me bound to the kitchen for hours. My meals are simple (anyone can prepare them), yet special.

I have discovered that "cooking" and "eating" are synonyms for "enjoying." We don't have to be at war with time and calories. It's important to enjoy yourself! Turn a daily task into a pleasure by cooking consciously. You're not just cooking, but creating, developing yourself, and feeding yourself and others. And when you use natural, high-quality ingredients, you know that every bite is good for you. You are free to enjoy your dinner without restricting portion sizes or counting calories.

How you eat is no less important than what you eat. I enjoy setting the table with beautiful plates, glasses, linens, and crafting a welcoming atmosphere—often outside. It's half the fun. I create my own beautiful world. That's why I started making my own dinnerware. I am a ceramist as well as an author. It gives me an immense feeling of satisfaction to make plates with my potter's wheel.

Healthy eating, for me therefore, has nothing to do with smoothies, juices, energy bars, and so on—where is the food, the pleasure? Where are the people? This so-called health food is far removed from real experiences. People think you can reduce food to a mere sum of vitamins and minerals. Where is the "true" life? For me, the act of eating itself is a source of happiness, a moment to be savored.

I hope this book will inspire you to try another way of eating. Forget calories, focus on quality, and let your body do the rest.

Love, Pascale

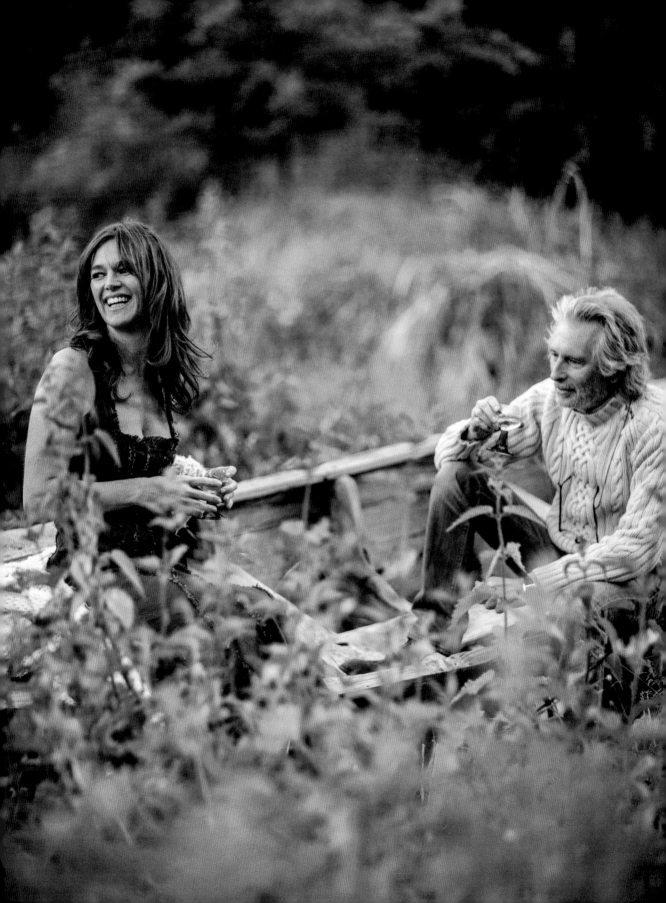

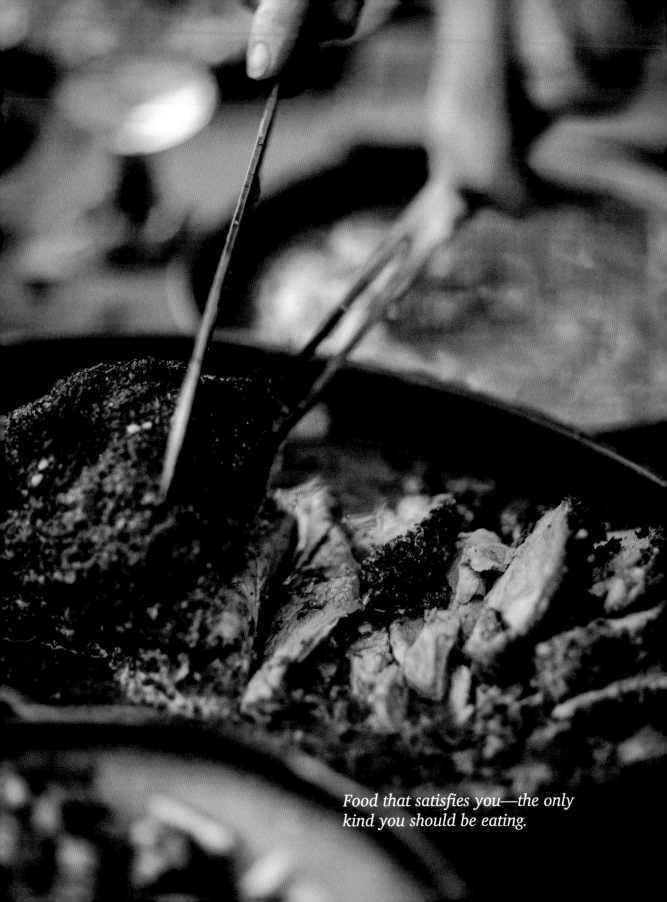

Food that satisfies you—the only kind you should be eating.

This Is Not a Diet. I Hate Diets.

In pages to follow, I answer questions that I have often received from readers and explain in detail my method of eating and the rationale behind it. But I think it's important to note that this is not a diet book. I hate diets because when I followed them, in the end they didn't work. The fight against extra pounds is always a losing fight. And willpower alone won't do it. This is why all diets fail. Good food, pleasure, and health—these are the most important aspects of my cooking. These terms may not automatically be associated with losing weight; however, people who are overweight lose weight when applying them, often to their own surprise. The only correct approach for everyone, thin or not, is to eat natural ingredients, food that gives you energy and a feeling of satisfaction. Eating natural foods will keep you healthy and slim. It will satisfy you. The craving for unhealthy comfort food and processed food will disappear.

If you want to successfully acquire new and healthy eating habits, there are two conditions:
– The food must be good.
– You must feel satisfied after each meal.

WILL I STILL ENJOY FOOD IF I EAT HEALTHY? WILL I BE HUNGRY?
These questions arise from an outdated vision of healthy nutrition. Many people think it is about eating less and eating food with less flavor (read: less fat). This vision also leaves us with guilt: If you gain weight, it is because you ate too many calories and then didn't burn them. Therefore, the culprit is you. Not enough willpower! But nothing is further from the truth. I eat much more than I used to; my food is more varied, more delicious, and contains more fat; I never eat "light" products; I don't count calories (that is so passé); I have a glass of wine; and I feel full after each meal. I freely enjoy my food; I never have any guilt, and still, I don't gain weight.

WHAT IS HEALTHY EATING?
The answer is actually very simple: eating natural food (see page 25 for a more detailed definition). This is nothing new: We all know that natural food is much healthier, but there is a huge difference between knowing and doing. This is why I have only one rule. By following this rule, you will eat differently, and the results will be amazingly good for your health . . .

MY ONE RULE: DO NOT EAT CONCENTRATED CARBOHYDRATES WITH CONCENTRATED PROTEIN IN THE SAME MEAL.

– Concentrated carbohydrates: bread, pasta, potatoes, rice, cereals, quinoa, buckwheat, beans, lentils, etc.
– Concentrated proteins: fish, meat, poultry, eggs, cheese, tofu, soy, seitan, shellfish, etc.

SO, YOU CAN EAT EVERYTHING,[1] BUT NOT TOGETHER.

When you eat like this, you have to make choices. Choose from among the following simple food combinations:

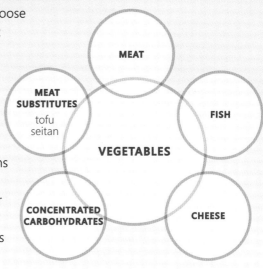

– fish + vegetables
– meat + vegetables
– eggs + vegetables
– cheese + vegetables
– carbohydrates + vegetables

So, in practice, following my rule of food combinations means nothing more than replacing things such as bread and potatoes with vegetables and fruits in your daily meals. Easy enough. But is it too good to be true and how do you make sure you are following this rule? Here are some more answers.

DON'T ALMOST ALL FOODS CONTAIN SOME PROTEIN AND SOME CARBOHYDRATES?

Yes, but I look at the *quantity* of carbs or protein in a particular food. I look at how much starch (carbohydrate) or protein there is in 100 grams of food. Anything that contains 10 grams of protein or more is classed as a protein. And anything containing 10 or more grams of starch is considered a carbohydrate. Concentrated carbohydrates have a high glycemic index or load, because they break down quickly during digestion. See page 19 for a more detailed discussion of carbohydrates. Vegetables, while they contain carbohydrates, are not considered concentrated and can be eaten with anything.

WHAT ABOUT FRUIT?

Fruit is not a concentrated carbohydrate, so it does not fall under the basic rule. However, fruit is a bit of a special case. When fruit ends up in a warm environment, such as the stomach, and cannot be digested quickly (for example, due to a full stomach), the fruit starts to ferment. Because many people suffer from this, it is better to eat fruit separately or eat it in a simple combination. For instance, mixing fruit with coconut milk is, of course, no

[1] Obviously I'm not talking about dessert and sweets.

problem; coconut itself is a fruit. Fruit also combines well with natural yogurt. For more on fruits, see page 182.

CAN I COMBINE DIFFERENT PROTEINS?

My basic rule is: Do not mix concentrated carbohydrates with concentrated proteins. I celebrate this rule and I will rarely deviate from it. I have selected the most important rule out of the food combining theory, but the traditional approach is much stricter than what I follow. For instance, mixing different kinds of protein is, I think, less important. There is, for now, no scientific consensus on this point.

My approach: I try to avoid combining different kinds of protein, because this makes for unnecessarily heavy meals. For example, meat and cheese. You will immediately notice that simple combinations improve digestion. While I prefer to combine eggs with vegetables, once in a while I combine them with cheese or meat. Or I use the yolk as a fat or condiment.

My advice is to test it yourself: How does it make you feel and what do you see on the scale?

WHAT ABOUT DAIRY?

Cheese: As mentioned above, cheese is a concentrated protein and is best combined with vegetables.

Milk: Many people have difficulties digesting cow's milk. Furthermore, many scientists don't recommend that adults drink milk for a variety of reasons. I do not use any milk in my recipes. I prefer coconut milk or almond milk. Soy milk is also okay if you like the taste.

Yogurt: Yogurt is quite healthy. It is a fermented product and promotes healthy bacteria in your gut. I always go for full-fat yogurt, never a light version. I combine yogurt with fruit in the morning. I rarely use it in other recipes because I love simple combinations, but feel free to eat it with everything. It is neither a concentrated source of protein nor a concentrated source of carbohydrates.

Cream: Heavy cream is mainly a source of fat, so you can combine it with everything. I see full-fat cream as a main ingredient, but not something that you put in every recipe. If I use cream, I use it for its flavor and its fat.

WILL I FEEL SATISFIED?

If you follow this rule, you will leave the table full and satisfied. It is wrong to think that carbohydrates are good "fillers." On the contrary, they are absolutely not. This is why you can so easily keep on eating them and overeat. The protein + fat + vegetable combination is the most satisfying. As you will see, I am not sparing with fat, but I am with carbohydrates. Fat not only provides flavor, but also makes you feel satisfied. The craving to eat more or to overeat disappears. Rest assured: You can help yourself to a double portion, preferably of vegetables, as long as you stick to the combinations.

WHAT ARE THE CONSEQUENCES OF THIS SINGLE RULE ON YOUR HEALTH?
Simple food combinations are digested more easily.
You will not suffer from a bloated stomach. Nutrients such as vitamins and minerals are not wasted: They are absorbed by the body, leaving you feeling fitter and healthier. We are the only beings on earth who eat everything together; moreover, we eat huge amounts of food (this is because the traditional Western diet is not satisfying). This weighs on the digestive system and slows it down; consequently, food begins to ferment and rot in your stomach and intestines, often resulting in bloating and cramping. In addition, this stimulates the growth of harmful bacteria in our gut, which can have a negative impact on our health (see Good Bacteria and Nutrition, page 176). Simple food combinations help your digestive system operate smoothly, without burden.

You will eat fewer unhealthy, addictive carbohydrates (potatoes, bread, pasta, rice, etc.).
Since you cannot eat concentrated carbohydrates with concentrated protein, you will not eat things such as bread or potatoes at every meal. Please note that you can still eat them, although only in combination with vegetables.

You will eat more vegetables.
If you eat less of potatoes and the like, you have to replace them with something else on your plate—vegetables. They form the basis of a healthy, energetic body.

If you are overweight, you will lose weight.
It has been proven that replacing potatoes and bread with vegetables during meals has a slimming effect. Not just because you're eating fewer carbohydrates, but also because this helps you eat the proper food combinations. Studies show that you will not gain weight by eating most kinds of proteins, such as fish, cheese, and eggs. They will even protect you against obesity. But when you eat these protein-rich foods combined with carbohydrates, such as potatoes or bread, it will be fattening. This was the conclusion of a recently published long-term study.[2]

[2] J.D. Smith, T. Hou, D.S. Ludwig, E.B. Rimm, W. Willett, F.B. Hu, and D. Mozaffarian, "Changes in intake of protein foods, carbohydrate amount and quality, and long-term weight change: results from 3 prospective cohorts," *The American Journal of Public Nutrition* (April 8, 2015).

YOU JUST NEED TO START.

I receive emails every day from women and men whose lives have changed dramatically after they began using my recipes. Recently, I talked with fifteen women whose lives had improved after they began using my recipes. They felt healthier and more energetic, and all of them had lost weight. In addition, they were unanimous about one thing: "It is so simple—you only need to make the switch."

THE HISTORY OF FOOD COMBINATION

The practice of not combining certain food groups and in particular not combining protein with carbohydrates has been around for a very long time. It was mentioned in the ancient texts of Tao Te Ching, which discussed wisdom, life, leadership, and health, in about the late fourth century BCE. Traditional Chinese medicine, one of the oldest forms of medicine, was based on these source books.[3] Avoiding combining certain food groups is a philosophy that has been handed down ever since and has always had a place in Asian folklore. Through the ages there have been groups of people that have applied this idea in different ways.

In the 1920s, the American physician Dr. William Howard Hay was one of the founders of the concept that became known as the "combination diet" or "separate nutrition." Throughout the world, enthusiastic nutritionists embraced the idea and began to see positive results in their patients. Since then, this method has been described in many popular books on health. The book *The Food Combining Diet*, by Kathryn Marsden, was published in 1993 and was a worldwide bestseller with more than seventeen reprints. The revised edition, *The Complete Book of Food Combining* (2005), is still selling consistently. This book is highly recommended if you would like to learn more about this topic.

A breakthrough in this regard was *Fit for Life*, by Harvey and Marilyn Diamond. This book was number one on bestseller lists worldwide for years. In Germany, they talk of *Trennkost*. The popular English foodie sisters Jasmine and Melissa Hemsley also take food combinations into account. Likewise, well-known American nutritionist Kimberly Snyder has inspired numerous American celebrities with her healthy combinations.

We cannot ignore the fact that food combining has become a worldwide phenomenon. It is a simple, safe way of eating; it has helped countless people improve their health. My husband and I have applied this method for over twenty years. I can only say this: You should simply try it!

---

[3] For a description of the history of food combination in relation to Taoism, see D. Reid, R. Munk, *De Tao van het lichaam: Een moderne, praktische benadering van een eeuwenoude levenswijze* (The Tao of the Body: A Modern, Practical Approach to an Age-Old Way of Life) (Amersfoort, the Netherlands: BBNC Uitgevers, 1999).

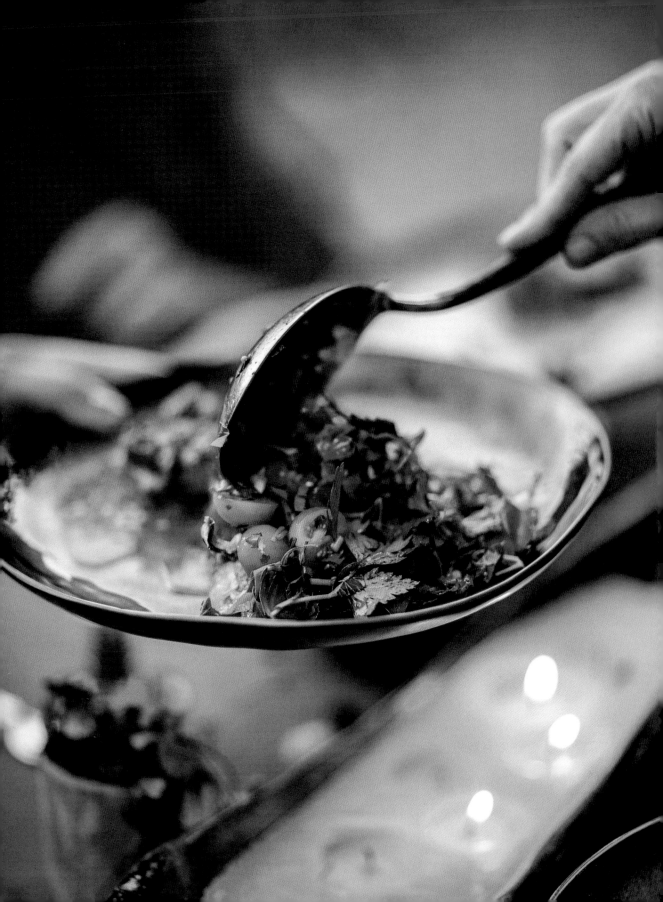

"Fast" versus "Slow" Carbohydrates

Since the term carbohydrate is used throughout this book, this section offers some further explanation of the role carbohydrates play in our diet. Also, I have a particular way of evaluating carbs and incorporating them in my meals that I'd like to share.

Carbohydrates can be found in many foods in varying degrees; they are actually chains of sugar molecules, like glucose, the smallest sugar molecule in our food.

The quality of the source of a carbohydrate is probably the most important thing to understand. The quality can be evaluated by the presence of fiber, nutrients, the glycemic response (the lower the better), and how heavily processed a carbohydrate is: Are the grains still intact or ground? Are you eating the fruit whole or is it pressed into juice?

You can use the glycemic index (or glycemic load) scale to calculate the rate at which carbohydrates are digested. Carbohydrates with a medium or low glycemic index or load are digested by the body more slowly, and these are considered to be healthier. "Fast" carbohydrates, or carbohydrates with a high glycemic index or load, on the other hand, are digested by the body more quickly and are considered less healthy.

The content of fiber and nutrients is also important. Natural sources of carbohydrates are often slow carbs. They are high in fiber and nutrients and include foods such as legumes, oats, wild and whole-grain rice, pseudo-grains like quinoa and buckwheat, whole grains like barley, most fruits, nonstarchy vegetables, and so on.

In contrast, processed, fast carbohydrates are lower in fiber and nutrients and higher in sugar. Fast carbohydrates include sugar, bread, potatoes, white rice, pasta, and so on. The digestion of these carbohydrates causes the release of a large amount of sugar, which can very quickly raise your blood sugar and insulin levels. This is unhealthy, and according to many scientists, it can cause obesity and type 2 diabetes.

I am not recommending that you cut out carbs, but rather be selective about the types you eat and what foods you combine them with.

GOOD SOURCES OF CARBOHYDRATES

I primarily replace potatoes, bread, pasta, and rice with vegetables and fruit.

What are the benefits?
– Vegetables and fruits contain fewer carbohydrates. And they are not fast carbohydrates.
– You will eat more fiber, vitamins, minerals, and other powerful antioxidants and phyto-chemicals that protect against various diseases.
– Vegetables and fruits are the healthiest types of food you can find; they are 100 percent natural and unprocessed.
– Vegetables and fruits are not addictive; you are unlikely to binge on or overeat these foods.

If I choose a meal with carbohydrates, I prefer:
– Pseudo-grains, such as buckwheat or quinoa;
– Legumes, such as chickpeas, lentils, or beans;
– Wild rice or brown rice; or
– Oatmeal.

These are all better suppliers of carbohydrates than refined starches, because:
– They are unrefined—less processed, transformed, or manipulated.
– They contain more fiber, so they release their sugar slowly and don't lead to a spike in your blood sugar. Fiber is also beneficial to your intestinal flora.
– They are more filling.
– They contain higher concentrations of vitamins, minerals, and amino acids.
– They are gluten-free.
– And perhaps most important, we have a tradition of preparing these kinds of foods in a healthy way.

MY DIET IS POOR IN "FAST" CARBOHYDRATES

At eighteen, I started dieting, and I struggled with my eating habits for years. There were periods when I had myself under control. I followed a diet based on calorie restriction out of pure willpower. However, I was always hungry; I became unhappy and could not keep it up. The result was that I had cravings for food and went through periods of binging when I only wanted one thing: fast carbohydrates. I don't know anyone who overeats fruit, fish, meat, or vegetables; I do know many people who binge on bread, fries, and breakfast pastries, though. All my weight and craving issues disappeared when I left the fast carbs behind and switched to pure, natural food.

EATING LESS CARBS AND MORE GOOD FAT

According to the classic nutritionist recommendation, we should be getting half to three-quarters of our daily energy from carbohydrates. However, emerging scientific views say that we don't need such high amounts of carbohydrates and that the conventional recommendations are actually the cause of obesity and diabetes epidemics. The classic recommendation was a lot of carbohydrates and little fat, while the new vision says the opposite—fewer carbohydrates and a reevaluation of good fats. This progressive nutritional vision is emerging everywhere in the world and gaining popularity. Well-known researchers and scientists are publishing numerous studies showing that fewer carbohydrates and more fat (especially olive oil) have positive effects on body weight, on the risk of diabetes and cardiovascular diseases, and on cholesterol levels.

I am not an expert, but I can speak from personal experience. I haven't eaten fast carbohydrates for over twenty years and I have had no problems with weight or addictive eating habits. I have a lot of energy and my doctor has been praising my excellent blood test results for many years. It is the same for my husband. On paper, and for some people, a lot of carbs may be okay, but for me and for so many others, they are a serious problem. My body cannot handle a large quantity of fast, refined carbohydrates. In the past, I got caught in their trap because they are very addictive. I became dependent on them and my hormones ran wild. Many people experience the same pitfalls.

I think the best way of eating is to keep a healthy balance of fats, protein, and good sources of carbs. This way of eating has made me feel great for years and the same is true for the many people who have changed the way they eat to reflect this new approach. Many email me to tell me how their energy levels have risen and how they have effortlessly lost weight. I often read: "This way of eating is easily sustainable." Readers also report a positive effect on chronic ailments such as high cholesterol, type 2 diabetes, gastrointestinal disorders, chronic fatigue syndrome, rheumatic disorders, and more.

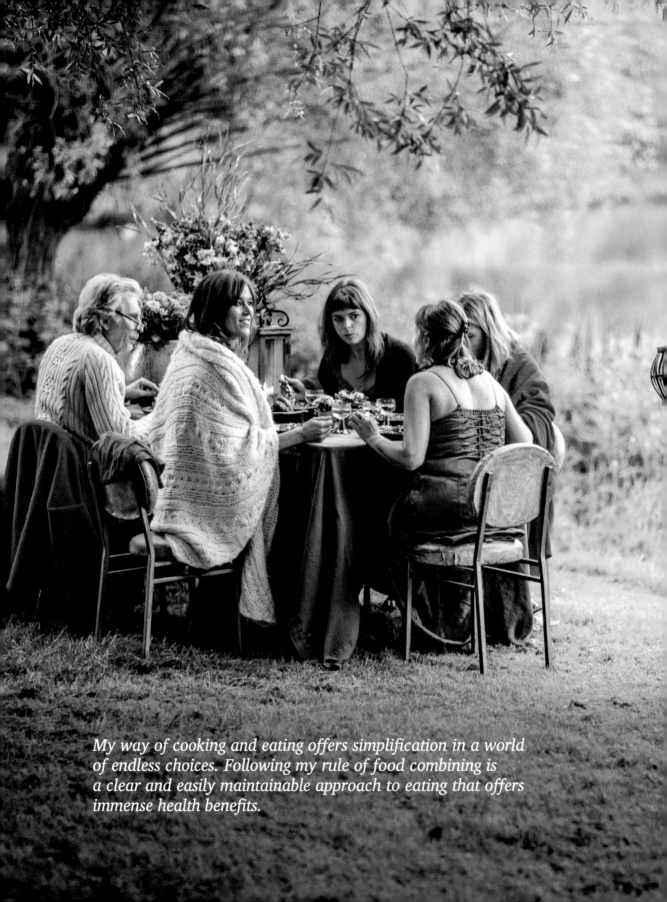

My way of cooking and eating offers simplification in a world of endless choices. Following my rule of food combining is a clear and easily maintainable approach to eating that offers immense health benefits.

What Should We Eat Tonight?

Name anything that grows, crawls, or swims—in short, anything that is alive—and you can be assured that it is being eaten by someone, somewhere in the world. Worms, insects, fish eyes, guts, brains, frog legs—someone eats it! Humans are omnivores; and at first sight, this seems to be an advantage.

However, it doesn't help us at the supermarket—quite the contrary. There we have to choose from an abundant array of foods. We are asked to make choices at least three times per day. We are all familiar with this stressful dilemma: "What should we have for dinner?"

Not only do we eat everything, we also seem to lack discernment. Even fake food and chemically processed junk without any nutritional value make their way to our stomachs. Fast-food hamburgers, croissants with chemical additives, imitation fish, fluorescent candy. We are easy prey for the food industry.

One of the biggest problems is that we have strayed far away from the source of our nutrition. We lost interest in the story behind it, in the origin of our food, in the way it is made. Eating must be fast, convenient, and preferably cheap. And so, we are constantly cheated by some food producers. Think, for example, of truffle oil (flavored with a petroleum extract) or some Norwegian salmon (loaded with pesticides and antibiotics and quickly fattened with the wrong food), or processed meat (made from pieces of meat that are glued together). All these are readily consumed by the unsuspecting omnivore.

A large part of the food industry finds it very convenient that we are not concerned about what we eat. They have found it easy to fool most consumers. For years we have not been interested in honest products offered and prepared with care by farmers, fishermen, and craftsmen. Ignorance is probably the consumer's greatest problem. If we only knew what has happened to create the food that lands on our plates, we would probably make different choices. This is why awareness is so important. We should be concerned, and that requires courage. We must take this seriously; we must look for information. It is our right.

When you realize, day after day, how delicious, tasty, and satisfying natural food is, how it provides energy and how it makes you stronger and healthier, you will never want anything else.

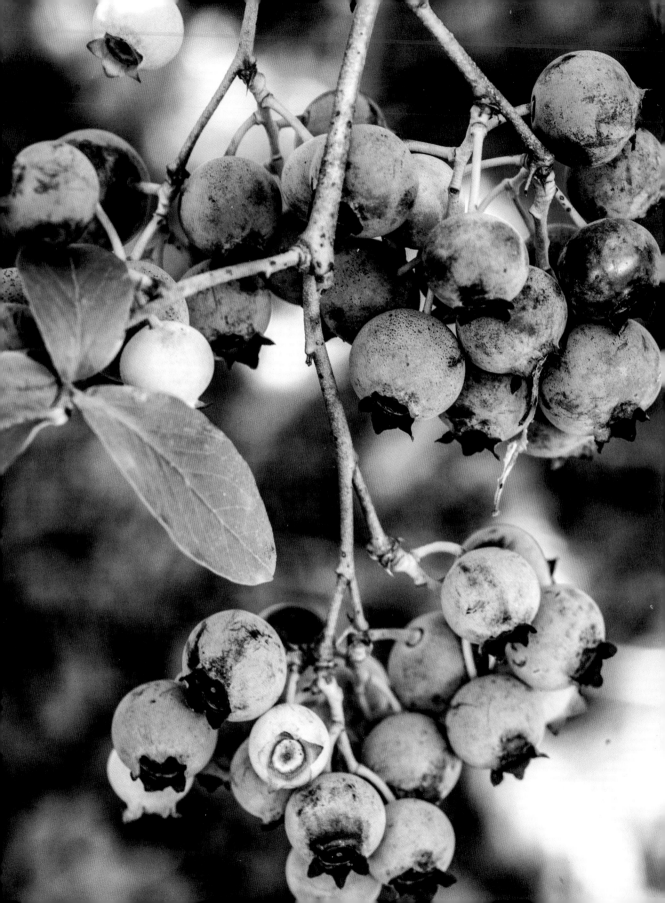

Natural Food Explained

Many people become overweight and sick because of what they eat. Every single day, newspapers publish information on nutrition and health. There are numerous theories and findings, almost all of which advocate the same thing: "Eat natural food."

But the problem is that we have forgotten what natural food is versus industrial or refined products. So, in this section I offer my explanation for how to identify natural foods and discuss some of the reasons to avoid processed foods.

Natural food grows on trees or shrubs; it comes out of the ground; it is living matter. This food is produced by nature. This food is not processed. It goes directly from the supplier to the store—think of vegetables, fruit, herbs, eggs, nuts, seeds, fish, meat, and so on. Even though refined food also originates from nature, it is industrially processed before reaching our plate. In a supermarket, approximately 75 percent of all food is refined or processed: breakfast pastries, bread, industrially prepared meals, preserves in glass jars or cans, sodas, cookies, snacks, and so on.

A century ago, most of our food was still natural; with the mechanization of agriculture and industrialization of the food sector, most of our food is now refined and processed. At first, this appears to be progress. Indeed, busy people find it very convenient to reheat a ready-made pizza or a prepared meal. As consumers, we have been exposed to advertising from specific food industries for decades. They made us believe that their food is the same as natural food, or even better. Nothing is further from the truth. Margarine is not natural fat. Industrial bread is not the same as whole-grain bread from the bakery. A package of sweet cookies is not healthy food, even if it says "high fiber" in big letters.

Refined food is not fulfilling; it has lost much of its valuable nutrition. You can never eat enough of it to be satisfied, and it is addictive. The only thing it provides is a lot of empty calories that make you fat and unhappy. I speak from experience because I was once addicted to this kind of food. Or, as doctor William Cortvriendt writes in his book, "Our body is not equipped with detectors that can correctly assess the nutritional value, or rather harm, of chemically produced foods."[4] The most powerful proof that refined food is not good for us is that it makes us fat. This is not related to our willpower or genes; nobody is immune to this type of food. Switch to natural food and you will instantly feel a difference.

---

[4] William Cortvriendt, *Living a Century or More: A Scientifically Fact-Based Journey to Longevity* (North Charleston, SC: CreateSpace Independent Publishing Platform, 2013).

If you eat more natural foods, you will immediately notice your body react—you have more energy, you never leave the table hungry, because natural food is satisfying; it puts you in a good mood, and it is infinitely more delicious than refined food.

FALSE FOODS

Fake food is deliberately made with large quantities of sugars, fats, and salt, so that they can provide the strongest possible stimulation to the primitive areas of the brain that play a role in pleasure and addiction.

—KRIS VERBURGH, *THE FOOD HOURGLASS*[5]

Processed fats, refined carbohydrates, and other drastically transformed foodstuffs manage to bypass our natural satisfaction mechanisms. As a result, we never feel full, and so we carry on eating. Just think of pasta, white bread, breakfast muffins, cookies, or chips—they are all things that are so easy to eat too much of. Perhaps the development of such foods was well intentioned at the time, but it is now clear that natural food products are much better for our health. Natural foods are full of important nutritional elements that can be both identified and absorbed by our body. In contrast, most industrial foodstuffs contain:
– hidden sugars or synthetic sweeteners;
– chemical substances, such as artificial colorants;
– preservatives;
– manipulated fats and trans fats; and
– too much salt.

What's more, the drastic preparation processes to which processed foods are subjected usually result in the most important nutritional elements being lost. In other words, they are an assault on our health.

It is now clear that good-quality butter, for example, is much healthier than margarine; that extra-virgin oil is much healthier than refined oil; that meat from animals raised in natural conditions is much healthier than meat from industrial farm-raised animals. Other research has shown that fructose in its natural environment—for example, in fruit—is health-giving, but that extracted fructose—in other words, removed from its natural environment—is not. The best sources of omega-3s continue to be walnuts, linseed, algae, fatty fish, and the red meat of animals fed on grass. These sources most certainly do *not* include food products "enriched" with omega-3s.

The food industry can do its best to try and make up for the loss of nutritional elements caused by its manufacturing processes, but at the end of the day a natural product will still have far more to offer in health terms than a man-made variant. The vitamin C in an

[5] Kris Verburgh, *The Food Hourglass: Stay Younger for Longer and Lose Weight* (London: HarperCollins, 2014).

orange is much better absorbed by the body when you eat the whole fruit than when you take an equivalent amount of vitamin C as a supplement.

Food producers have a tendency to alter food to meet their own needs and requirements—or at least they try. But why?
– To make food sweeter and more attractive, so that they can sell more of it.
– To prolong the sell-by and use-by dates.
– To increase production, because economies of scale mean more profit and lower prices.

WHAT TO AVOID
Healthy eating is actually very simple—just eat natural foods. So, the following products and ingredients should be avoided:

Refined Oils
The refinement process makes possible a significant increase in oil yield. But the severe nature of the refining (at very high temperatures or with the use of chemical solvents) means that most of the important nutrients in the oils are lost. All that remains is "unnatural" oil that is harmful to our health.

Store-Bought Mayonnaise
How many ingredients do you need to make mayonnaise? Four: oil, eggs, mustard, and lemon juice. But look at the list of ingredients on the bottle of mayonnaise that you buy at your local supermarket. You will find modified starch, sugar, preservatives, and more.

Fruit Drinks
Sugars in a soluble state (for example, in sodas, but also in fruit drinks) are absorbed much faster than in their natural state (in other words, as found in the fruit itself). For this reason, it is much better to eat fruit than to drink fruit drinks. Fast sugars cause high blood sugar spikes, which are not good for our health. Our stomachs are full, but almost half of us are suffering from a deficiency in important vitamins and minerals.

White Flour
White flour is used to make, among other things, white bread and cookies. In other words, our convenience foods. You can regard it as grain that has been ruined. Everything good and healthy has been removed: the germ, bran, much of the fiber, and also the nutrients. All that remains is an energy-compact foodstuff with no added nutritional value. In fact, it has been shown in recent years that this "foodstuff" can actually make you ill.

Trans Fat
In order to transform highly fluid oils, such as corn oil or sunflower oil, into more viscous forms of fat, they are subjected to a severe process known as hydrogenation or the

hardening of the fats. This results in the creation of unnatural trans fatty acids that are very bad for our health. Unfortunately, these are very cheap oils for the food industry to work with. So, they are used for the industrial manufacture of cookies, cakes, and deep-fried foods, such as potato chips and French fries. "Trans fatty acids are unhealthy, put extra stress on the heart and arteries, upset the healthy working of the nervous system and encourage inflammation. Consuming 5 grams of trans fatty acids per day increases the risk of cardio-vascular disease by 25 percent."[6]

Skimmed or Fat-Free Dairy Products

Another good example of food manipulation is described by Michael Pollan in his book on real food.[7] In order to make dairy products low-fat, it is not sufficient simply to remove the fat content. It is necessary to apply a number of other processes so that the milk remains "creamy." This usually means that milk powder is added. But milk powder contains oxidized cholesterol, which, according to scientists, is worse for our arteries than ordinary cholesterol. What's more, the removal of the fat from the milk makes it more difficult for your body to absorb fat-soluble vitamins—the vitamins that are one of the main reasons for drinking milk in the first place!

Industrially Produced Proteins

Even a seemingly natural food like beef or fish can be unhealthy if produced with industrialized methods. Michael Pollan has asked whether the meat of a cow that has never been allowed to graze in natural surroundings, but has been fed exclusively on corn, cereals, concentrates, hormones, and antibiotics, can actually be regarded as a "natural" product. Unlike a cow that is raised on soy and corn, a cow raised on a diet of grass and other greens produces high levels of omega-3 fatty acids in its milk and meat. According to Professor Muskiet, the same is true for farmed fish (salmon, trout, tilapia, and so on) in comparison to wild fish.[8]

IT'S TIME TO HARNESS THE POWER OF NATURAL FOOD

It is the interaction of all its different nutritional elements that makes a natural food so powerful and health-giving. Science has the knowledge to break down a foodstuff into its different component parts, but creating a new nutritional product from scratch is much more difficult—if not impossible.

We need to have more respect for nature and for ourselves. Above all, we must not forget that we are a part of nature as well. Over the years, we have exchanged our natural foods for highly processed substitutes, but we now need to reverse this process—and fast!

[6] Annik Mollen. Kerngezond: *Biofysisch evenwicht voor een optimaal celmilieu* (In Perfect Health: Biophysical Balance for Optimal Cell Environment) (Leuven, Belgium: Lannoocampus, 2012).
[7] Michael Pollan, *In Defense of Food: An Eater's Manifesto* (New York: Penguin, 2008).
[8] Frits Muskiet is a professor of chemistry, medical nutrition, dietetics, and physiology at the University of Groningen.

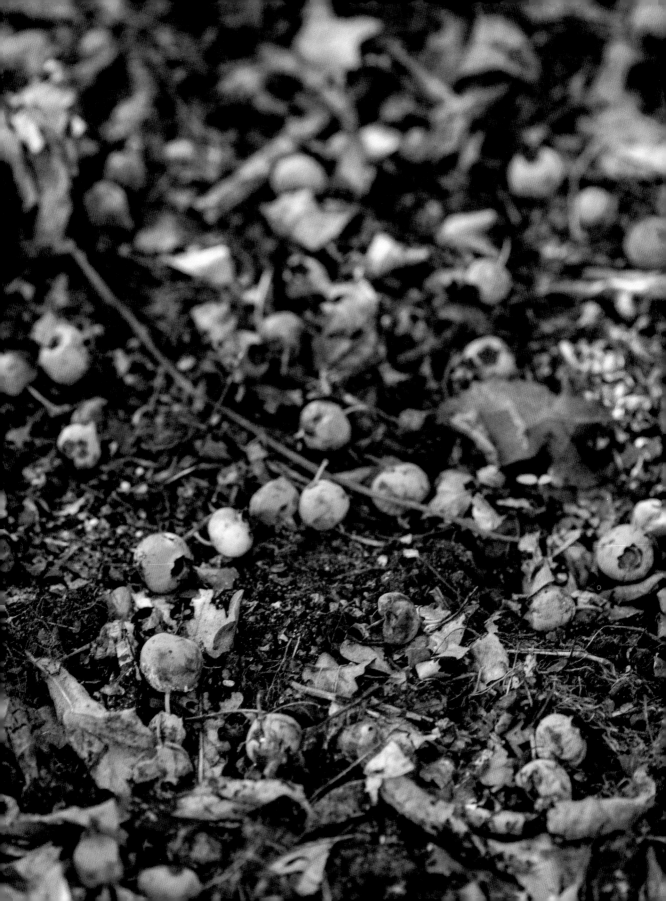

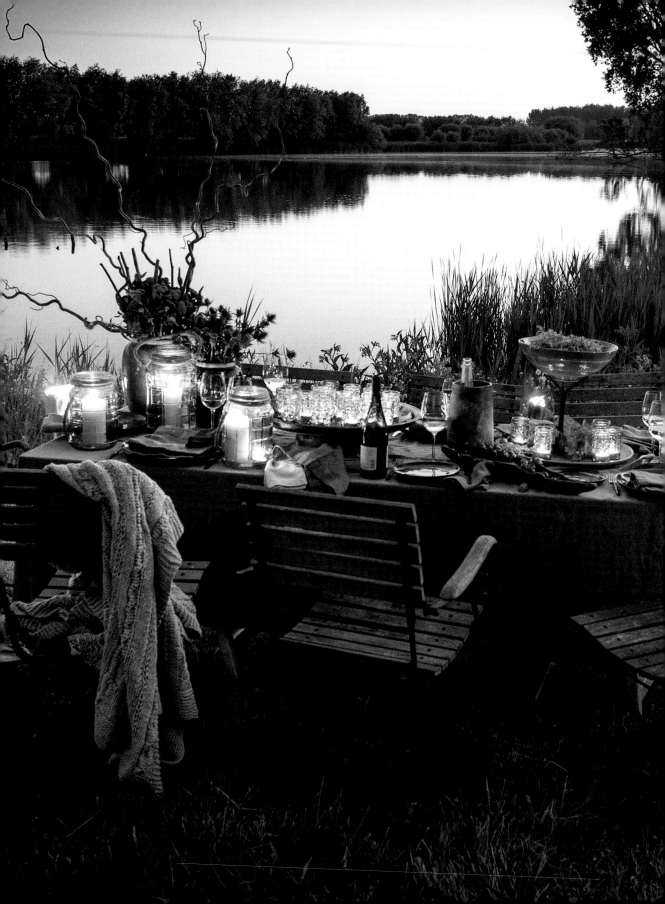

How to Use My Book

QUANTITIES ARE NOT IMPORTANT; EAT UNTIL YOU FEEL SATISFIED

Ideally, I would write recipes without specifying quantities or serving sizes. Some people need more calories than others, depending on their level of activity, gender, age, metabolism, and so on. However, portions also vary depending on whether you serve a dish separately or as part of a menu. Basically, there is only one single rule: Nobody leaves the table hungry! Eat until you have had enough. Take a double serving, preferably of vegetables, don't be sparing on fat and always respect the simple combinations. Protein satisfies immediately, fat is satisfying in the long run, and vegetables give volume. The protein + vegetables + fat combination satisfies much more effectively than a mountain of fast carbohydrates such as potatoes, pasta, or bread.

KEEP THESE BASIC INGREDIENTS IN STOCK

I assume that you always have the following basic ingredients in your kitchen; therefore, they are not included in the recipe ingredient lists:
– Extra-virgin olive oil
– Salt
– Black pepper (freshly ground)

KNOW YOUR OVEN

A wide range of ovens are available. In a conventional oven, radiant heat emanates from an element at the top and/or at the bottom of the oven. A convection oven uses a fan to circulate hot air throughout, which allows for faster preheating and cooking times. The times and temperatures stated in this cookbook are designed for convection ovens. For those who have conventional ovens, either increase the temperature by about 25 degrees or extend the baking time slightly. For example, 350°F (180°C) in a convection oven = 375°F (190°C) in a conventional oven. Keep in mind that the stated temperatures and cooking times are not exact and are dependent on the quantity of food, the material and shape of the baking dish, the oven, kitchen temperature, and so on. I recommend testing your oven to make sure the temperature gauge is accurate and also periodically checking your food while it is baking. My recipes include information on how you can make sure your food is baked to perfection.

SEEK BALANCE

Healthy eating is not about radical choices; on the contrary, it is about finding the right balance. I used to find this rather boring; now I know it is a beautiful and powerful story. Nature strives for balance: It is about harmony, and harmony brings peace. Ever since I found the right balance in my eating habits, I actually have the feeling that I can eat anything and that I am much freer in my choices.

However, nutrition is not the only important thing; exercise is also a necessary component of a healthy lifestyle. And of course how you live your life: how you deal with stress, how much you enjoy your day-to-day activities. All these factors are essential to your health, and in large part they are in your own hands. Get started, and integrate new habits and insights in your life, step by step.

EXERCISE

This book is essentially about nutrition, but I find exercise at least as important. First, I never choose the easiest way: I take the stairs (even if there is an elevator); I park my car far away from the door; I sit as little as possible. Every day, I try to have a "conscious exercise moment." It gives me peace of mind and keeps my body flexible. Yoga is a good example. I admit that I thought yoga was nothing but hype when I first tried it while on vacation. Now I understand why so many people are devoted to it. My husband, Paul, and I are convinced. Not a day goes by without a yoga moment for me. I can truly recommend it to anyone: young, old, stiff, or limber . . . it can be beneficial to anyone. Besides yoga, walking is my favorite exercise. It can be a thirty-minute brisk walk or a longer weekend stroll for a couple of hours. It calms my mind; every time, I am amazed at the beauty of nature. It makes me happy.

CAN I *THIS* OR CAN I *THAT*?

Nothing in life is black or white; our diet certainly isn't. I want to enjoy life; I don't want to exclude anything. A little "bad" eating will not hurt us; moreover, if you really savor and appreciate the occasional decadent food, then the fight is almost won, since it means that you have a conscious approach to nutrition. I believe that 70 to 80 percent of what you eat must be "real" food. Obviously, this means food that has nutrients to offer your body, foods like vegetables, fruit, nuts, grains, fish, meat, and eggs. The remaining 20 or 30 percent can be what I call "comfort food": dessert, fries, bread, candy, and so on. This proportion will make you a happy and healthy person.

Simply use your common sense and know which foods you should eat in large quantities and which foods you should eat sparingly. For instance, I eat a piece of chocolate every day with my green tea. Everybody has weaknesses, and that is a good thing.

HAVE DESSERT

Eating an occasional dessert cannot hurt you; on the contrary, this is food for the soul. Don't even try to find healthy desserts. Desserts are almost always unhealthy. If I eat dessert, I choose the true, full delicacy—certainly not the light version. I feel fulfilled, both mentally and physically, and the craving disappears. No need for large portions—on the contrary. Give dessert the value it deserves, but as an extra, something exceptional, reserved for special occasions. You will enjoy it even more.

SNACKS: YES OR NO?

My ideal snacks are nuts. Fresh fruit and unsweetened full-fat yogurt are also okay. However, only eat snacks if you are really hungry, not as occupational therapy. Did you know that your stomach and small intestine are self-cleaning? However, they can only clean themselves when digestion is fully completed.[9] Somebody who eats constantly never gives his stomach and small intestine the time to clean themselves.

WHAT ABOUT DRINKS?

Drink when you are thirsty. Water is the healthiest drink for humans. One advantage of a fruit breakfast (see page 182) is that it increases your fluid intake. Other preferred drinks for me are herbal tea (I especially like mint tea) and all green tea variations. Not only are they delicious, but they are also very healthy. Water, tea, and, every once in a while, a little champagne—these are my drinks. Try to avoid sweetened or diet sodas.

WHAT ABOUT ALCOHOL?

In limited quantities, alcohol is not harmful to the liver; it is perfectly capable of processing alcohol. The problem is quantity: The available enzymes in the liver are insufficient to process a lot of alcohol.

Many studies show that a limited amount of alcohol actually has a protective effect against cardiovascular diseases. Red wine has a small advantage thanks to the presence of polyphenols. Therefore, moderate drinking offers advantages; however, if you drink more than your liver can handle, all the positive aspects will be reversed and alcohol becomes very toxic and extremely harmful to your health. New research shows a strong link between alcohol and breast cancer, so women especially have to be careful. Enjoying a good-quality wine once in a while will allow you to enjoy the pleasant effects of alcohol, personally and socially. If you can't limit your drinking, you should avoid alcohol altogether.

[9] Giulia Enders, *Gut: The Inside Story of Our Body's Most Underrated Organ*, Vancouver: Greystone Books, 2015.

GO GROCERY SHOPPING

My dishes are very simple, easy, and quick to prepare. However, grocery shopping does take time, because I only use fresh, natural ingredients. We often consider grocery shopping to be a chore, which is a shame. Indeed, this means that we aren't prioritizing quality food and that we aren't acknowledging how important nutrition is to our health. I say this often: You don't need to eat healthier for me; you must only do it for yourself because it will make you a better person. If you accept this premise, you will find shopping for groceries and preparing meals to be well worth the time involved. It begins with love and respect for yourself.

BUY THE BEST INGREDIENTS YOU CAN FIND

It is true that healthy food is more expensive. This is a pity, although we do have a choice: Either we pay the price with our health and eventually spend more on doctor's appointments and medications, or we pay the price for quality food. These foods make your body strong, slim, and healthy and help you to enjoy a long, vigorous life.

Why shouldn't we spend our money on quality food if it helps to keep us healthy?

Buy the best ingredients you can find. Go for quality. Be proud of your ingredients. If possible, buy directly from the farmer or the fisherman. Know where your food comes from. Quality has a price; however, you will be plentifully rewarded in the form of an energetic, strong, and healthy body. Really—what is true wealth in life?

DON'T BE TOO HARD ON YOURSELF

In the beginning, switching to healthier eating is an effort; it requires determination. However, you will be greatly rewarded. I encourage you to gradually integrate new habits into your existing diet. Every step is a step forward. The physical changes you experience—more energy, a firmer body—will encourage you to progress on the path you have chosen. Don't be too strict, and don't blame yourself when something doesn't work. Most importantly, don't fight yourself. Listen to your body, listen to your gut, and find the harmony in yourself. Then it will feel like a natural process.

GET MOTIVATED

I don't want to convince you; I want to inspire you. Freedom is the most precious thing to have in life. It allows everyone to eat as he or she wants. I am the last person for whom you need to eat healthier. You must do it only for yourself. Making the changes has to be your choice, or you won't reach your health goals. Because you bought this book, however, I suspect you have already made your decision and that you are already interested in the wonderful world of natural food. I can only hope that my enthusiasm is infectious, because I am highly convinced that food makes a difference. I have experienced it firsthand, and I keep feeling it every day.

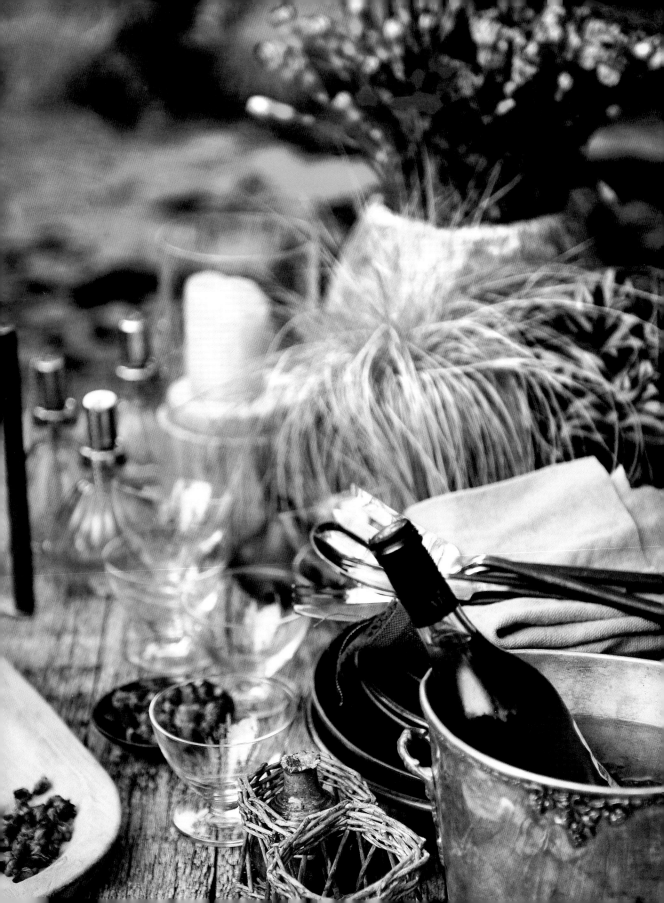

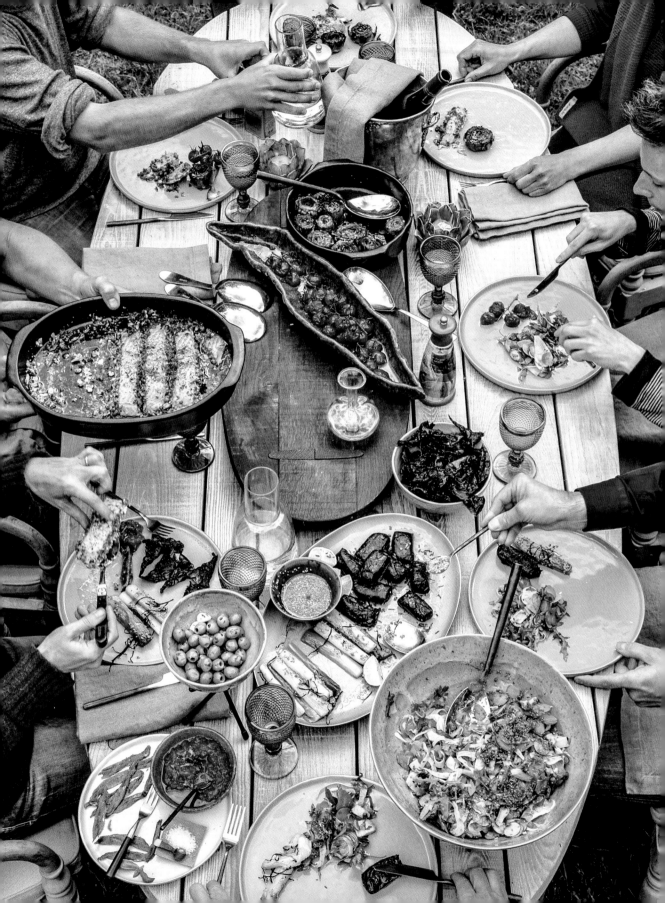

Mix and Match My Recipes to Create Rich, Original Meals

My recipes are not meant to be primarily used as standalone lunches or dinners. When friends come over, I like to serve all sorts of different dishes at the same time—while still following the rules of food combining. I cover my table with an assortment of delicious, colorful dishes that I present in my most beautiful bowls and plates. It is a relaxed and fun way to entertain. Everyone can take what and as much as they want, which creates a pleasant buzz around the table. Your guests will enjoy the varied, wonderful fragrances, colors, and flavors. And this is also great for you as the host or hostess—there is no issue with plate order or timing. All the work is in the preparation, and once your guests arrive, you can simply enjoy the meal.

ONE OF MY FAVORITE MENUS
Salmon with Olive-Pistachio Tapenade and Tomatoes (page 66)
Fish Wraps with Sesame-Soy Dipping Sauce (page 78)
Avocado, Fennel, Carrot, and Radish Salad with Marinated Sesame
    Seeds (page 173)
Baked Artichokes (page 162)
Anchovies with Tomato Tartare (below)

Anchovies with Tomato Tartare

SERVES
4

PREPARATION
7 minutes

COOKING TIME
none

6 ripe tomatoes

10 anchovy fillets

Cut the tomatoes into quarters. Remove the seeds and cores.

Flatten the tomatoes and cut the skin off. Cut the flesh into cubes or pulse once or twice in a food processor (but do not blend excessively—you don't want to puree the tomatoes into a sauce). Transfer to a bowl and add a little olive oil, salt, and pepper. Put the tomatoes on a small serving plate and put the anchovies on top.

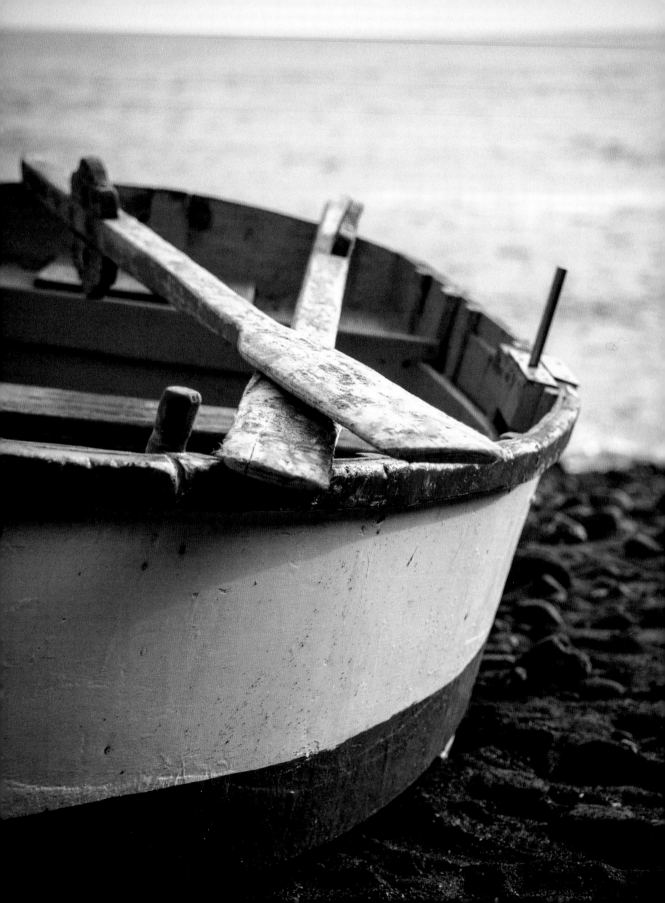

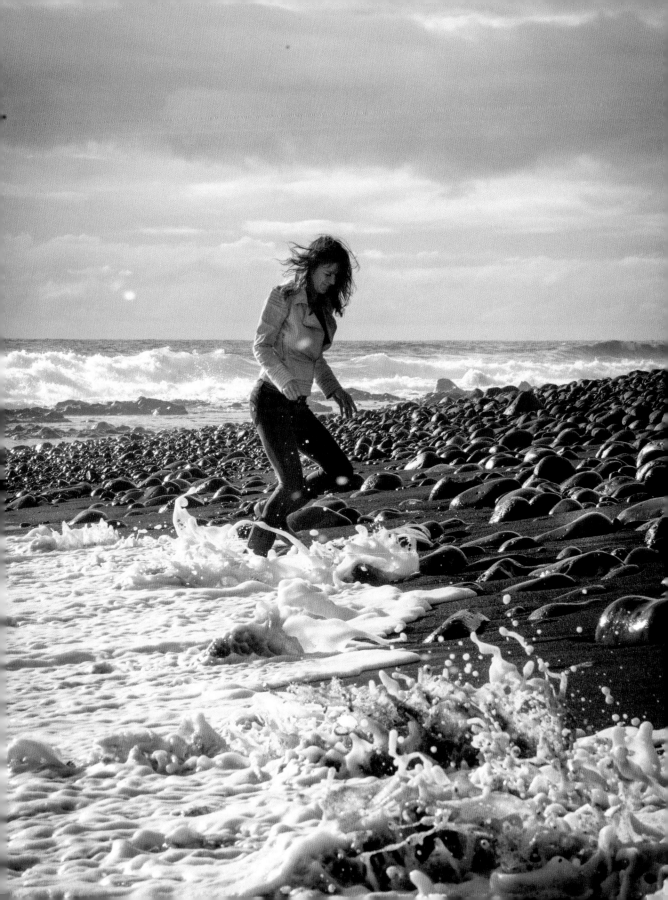

The Waterfront, Source of All Life

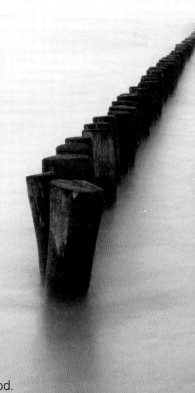

I heard the term "land-water ecosystem" for the first time when interviewing Dutch professor Frits Muskiet. He talked about human evolution and claimed that we probably originated from this ecosystem. He also addressed the topic of nutrition: Food that man would find along the coast—fish, shellfish, and marine plants—may be at the root of our brain growth. It is truly "brain food."

There are several different theories on the exact trajectory of human evolution—we don't know exactly how it happened. The most common theory is that our herbivorous ancestors came out of the forest and spread out throughout the vast savannah, becoming skillful hunters in the process; however, this theory has been increasingly questioned by scientists. They have identified one element that was essential to our development—water. According to these researchers, our ancestors lived mostly along the water—lakes, seas, and rivers—because it was a constant, reliable source of food.

The waterfront has always had a particularly powerful attraction for me. I spent my childhood on the banks of a creek in the beautiful lowlands of the Flemish coast. I enjoy diving, sailing, swimming, and fishing, and I like to walk along the Zeeland coast in the Netherlands, where you can still find oysters, seaweed, and marine plants. And if you go a little deeper into the water, you can see crabs and lobster (although if you try to harvest them, you will get a hefty fine!).

Where there is water, there is life. Some of the largest, deepest lakes in the world are located in central Africa, where some of the earliest humans developed. I find very plausible the theory that men went inland to hunt while women gathered everything edible, such as plants, berries, shellfish, fish, sea plants, eggs, and tubers.

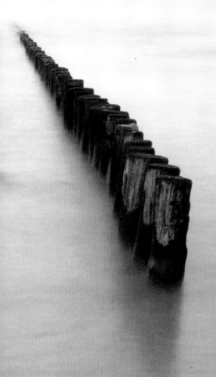

Researcher Remko Kuipers is a supporter of this theory. It is no coincidence that I asked him to write the foreword (see page 6) of this volume. In his own book *Het oerdieet* (*The Primal Diet*), Kuipers refers to British scientist Michael Crawford, who demonstrated the relationship between the amount of omega-3 fatty acids in the human diet and the dramatic increase in the size of the human brain throughout evolution. He explains that these omega-3s essentially come from fish, algae, and seaweed. These seafoods and plants also contain important substances essential for the development of the brain: iodine, selenium, and zinc. Crawford and other scientists have concluded that at least part of the food of our ancestors must have originated in the water.

The shift from a nearly vegetarian diet, such as that eaten by chimpanzees, to a complex diet that included more proteins and fats—fish, plants, meat, nuts, seeds, and poultry—proved to be essential for our brain growth. In addition, the discovery of fire, used to heat the food, making it more digestible and convertible into energy, was an important step in our development to *Homo sapiens*.

Over a period of a few million years, the human brain size increased dramatically. This was a very slow process. The idea that our ancestors, with their still very small brains, would have wandered into the savannah to hunt dangerous animals, such as buffalo and wildebeest, is hard to imagine. They did not yet have the intelligence to develop inventive hunting techniques. With a lot of luck, they could probably catch small game and birds. Some scientists conclude that man began to hunt buffalo and other large game much later, after the development of the brain. Moreover, research shows that the hunter-gatherer, even with a larger brain, was not a very successful hunter and often came home empty-handed. This theory suggests that man is not as great a meat eater as was initially thought. This, again, is consistent with current studies that show that eating too much red meat is unhealthy.

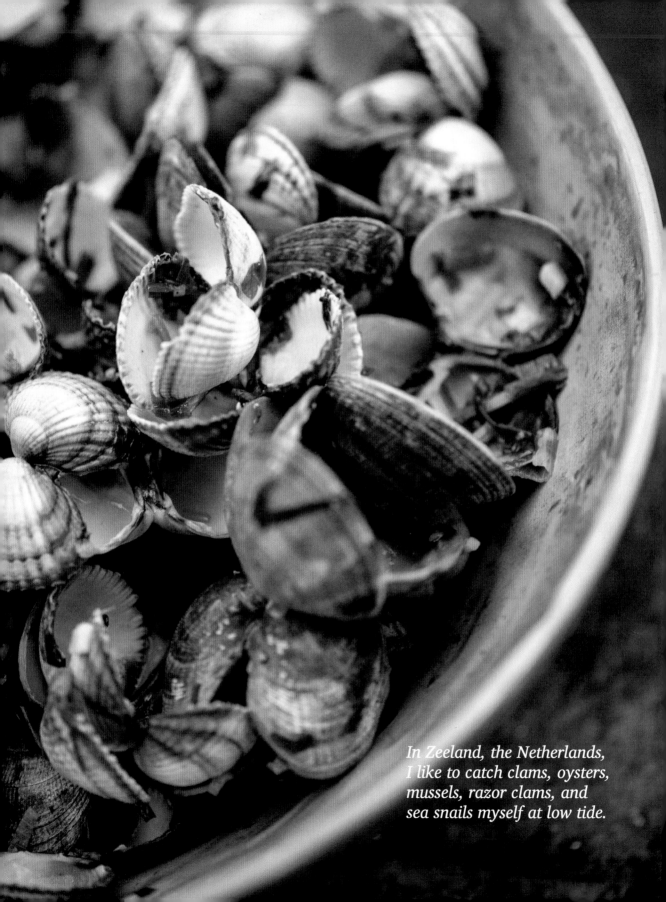

*In Zeeland, the Netherlands,
I like to catch clams, oysters,
mussels, razor clams, and
sea snails myself at low tide.*

Water has always been a compelling force in our history. It is no coincidence that many of our greatest cities were built along the water. The most fertile soil is found where land and water meet. And so, food rich in nutrients can be found in these areas—fish, shellfish, and seaweed from the water's edge; sheep, goats, and cows that graze in the nearby fields; fruits, vegetables, and herbs that grow along rivers. Water is life.

There is another reason why I believe in this theory of our evolution near the water: Today, the natural foods commonly found in these areas are considered to be elements of the healthiest diet—lots of vegetables, fruit, herbs, nuts, seeds, fish, shellfish, and, every once in a while, a little meat.

I love life along the waterfront—and the delicacies that this ecosystem has to offer. I love walking along the creeks, sometimes sitting in fields among sheep and cows for a picnic. On the coast, I like to search for seaweed, oysters, and shellfish. At night, I have gone along with North Sea fishermen to catch shrimp. In the polders, I can find all sorts of delicious vegetables and fruits. I'm always in search of "real" food—pure food that gives you energy and makes you strong. However, eating is not my only source of happiness.

Spending time in this powerful, beautiful natural setting brings joy. Bonding with the sources of my nutrition makes me happy. And so for me, all the puzzle pieces of living well—with happiness and health—come together in this book. Here I share my love of seafood and life near the water, my method of food combination, my celebration of natural foods, and the recipes that make improving your health not only easy but a pleasure.

SOURCES

Geoff Bailey and Nicky Milner. "Coastal Hunter-Gatherers and Social Evolution: Marginal or Central?" *Before Farming* 3–4, no. 1, January 2002.

Stephen C. Cunnane. *Survival of the Fattest: The Key to Human Brain Evolution*. Singapore: World Scientific Publishing Company, June 2005.

Remko Kuipers. *Het oerdieet: Dé manier om oergezond oud te worden* (The Paleo Diet: The Only Way to Healthy Aging). Amsterdam: Bert Bakker, 2014.

Heather Pringle. "Did Humans Colonize the World by Boat? Research Suggests Our Ancestors Traveled the Oceans 70,000 Years Ago," *Discover*, June 2008.

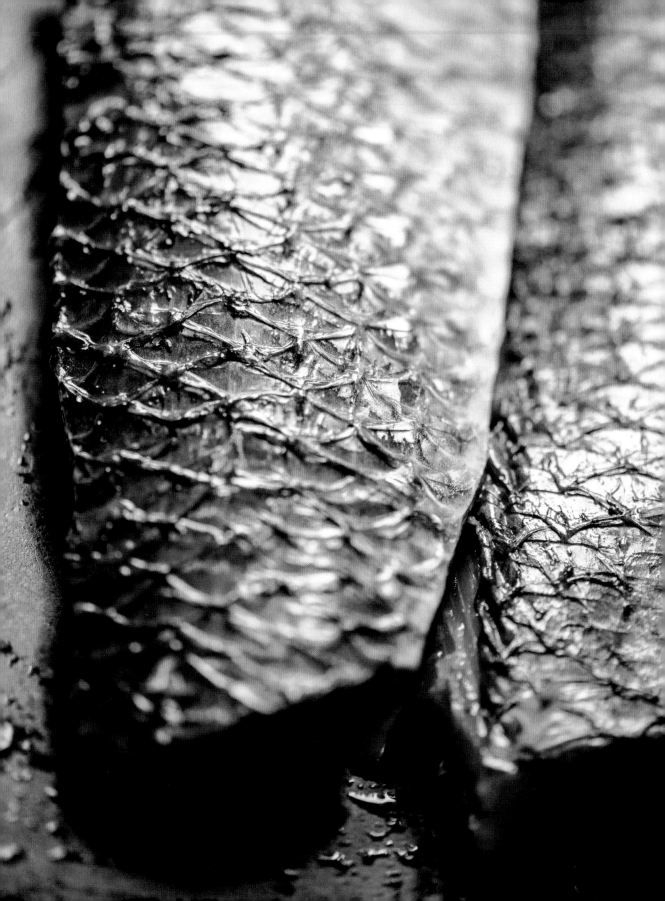

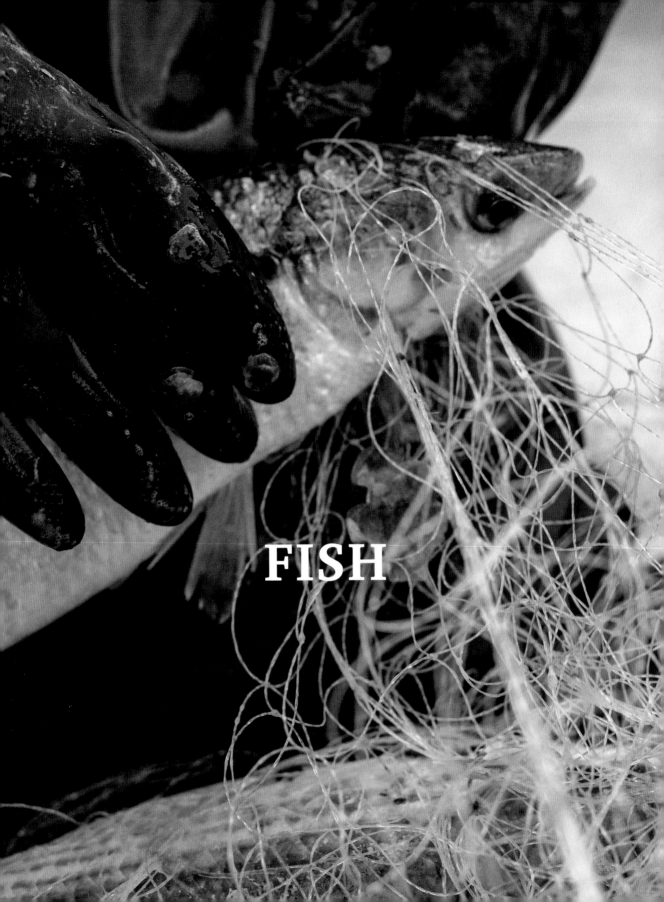

FISH

Cured Herring Tartare with Scallions

20 green beans

2 cured Dutch herring (maatjes; see tip)

2 scallions

1 bunch dill

Bring a medium saucepan of water to a boil and add a splash of olive oil. Add the beans and cook for 3 to 4 minutes, until just tender. Drain the beans and cool them under cold running water. Pat dry and cut them into small pieces. Season with salt and pepper.

Clean the herring with the dull side of a knife and cut them into small pieces. Finely chop the scallions and dill, reserving a small portion of dill for garnish.

Combine all the ingredients in a medium bowl and mix well. Place one ring mold on each of two plates and fill them with the mixture; press firmly, then remove the rings. Garnish with the reserved dill.

TIP: Maatjes

Maatjes are young herring. They are a fatty fish with a lot of flavor. Typically eaten in Belgium and the Netherlands, they are raw and brined. If you can't find them, look for other kinds of cured herring, not too sour or too sweet, or try this same preparation using raw salmon or tuna instead.

If you haven't tried cured herring, take a cue from the Belgians— this is a simple, delicious appetizer!

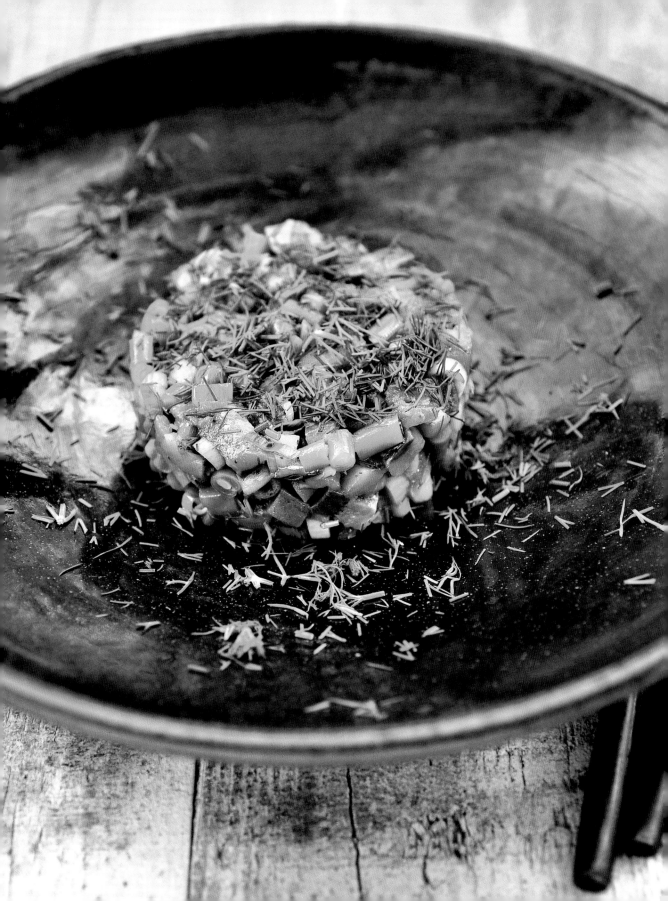

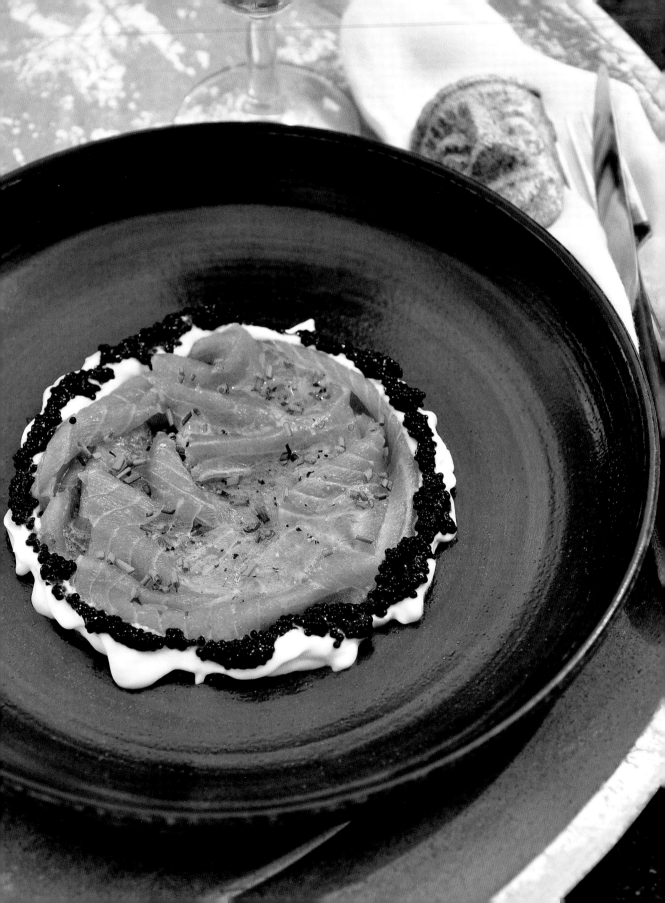

SERVES
4 as a light snack
or 2 as an appetizer

PREPARATION
10 minutes

COOKING TIME
none

Salmon Sashimi with Cream and Roe

7 ounces (200 g) raw salmon, sliced (see tip)

juice of 1 lemon

a few chive sprigs

3 or 4 tablespoons heavy cream

1 (2-ounce/57-g) jar lumpfish roe (see tip)

Divide the salmon among two or four plates, laying the slices in the center of the plates. In a small bowl, mix a dash of olive oil with the lemon juice and sprinkle this mixture over the salmon. Season with pepper and a little salt, and finish with some chopped chives.

In a bowl, whip the cream with an electric mixer until thick. Spoon the cream around the salmon and top with the roe. Serve immediately.

TIP: Salmon
Count on 1½ ounces (40 g) per person as a snack, or 3½ ounces (100 g) as a starter.

TIP: Lumpfish roe
Lumpfish roe is a more affordable version of caviar, and I love it. Real caviar comes from the sturgeon and is quite expensive. Lumpfish is a common fish typically found in the North Atlantic. The eggs are lightly salted, giving it a nice flavor. In fact, you could use any roe as long as it is real: I do not recommend imitation roe; its taste and texture are less appealing.

TIP: Combining heavy cream and protein
Full-fat cream is primarily a source of fat, and you can combine it with everything, including protein. I see cream as an essential main ingredient, playing a role like it does in classic French cuisine. It is not something that I would want to use in every dish, but I use it occasionally for its flavor and its fat.

I like to serve this for dinners that require a special touch. This is such an elegant but uncomplicated way to begin a meal.

MAKES
8 lollipops

PREPARATION
15 minutes

COOKING TIME
20 minutes

Sole Lemongrass Lollipops

1⅓ cups (40 g) coarsely chopped fresh herbs (see tip)

2 (9- to 11-ounce/255- to 310-g) sole, cut into 8 skinless fillets

8 lemongrass stalks

Preheat the oven to 350°F (180°C).

Finely chop the herbs. Place them in a bowl and mix them with a bit of salt, pepper, and olive oil.

Lay the sole fillets on your work surface with the side where the skin was facing down; sprinkle with the herbs. Set the tender end of one lemongrass stalk on each fillet and roll the fillet around the stalk like a lollipop (see tip). Set them upright (lemongrass "handles" sticking up) in a baking dish. Drizzle with olive oil and season with salt and pepper. Bake for 20 minutes.

TIP: Fresh herbs
Mix any herbs that you like: basil, flat-leaf parsley, cilantro, dill, and so on.

TIP: Rolling
It is important to roll the fillets so that the side where the skin was faces down. If you don't, they will unroll while cooking. Still, you may see one or two fillets unroll, but that won't be a problem. On the contrary, it makes the dish prettier and more creative.

TIP: Don't eat these with your hands
These rolled fillets are not intended to be eaten with your hands, even though it may be tempting. The sole does not remain tightly attached around the lemongrass, and parts will fall off. Save your guests from making a mess and serve the rolled sole fillets at the table with other dishes and vegetables so that guests can help themselves with utensils.

TIP: Lemongrass
Do not forget to chew on the lower part of the lemongrass, as it has a delicious, sweet lemon flavor.

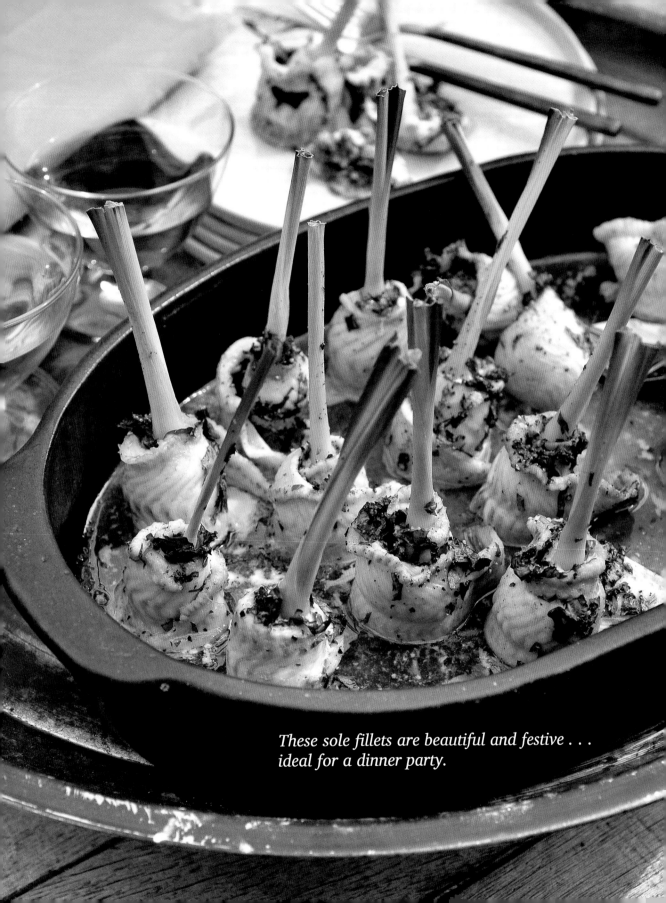

*These sole fillets are beautiful and festive . . .
ideal for a dinner party.*

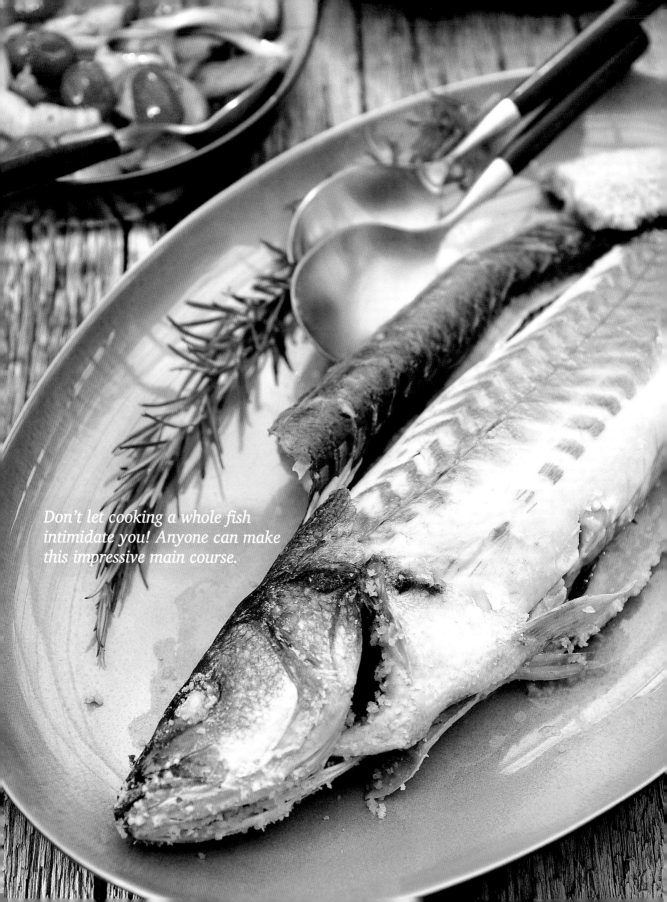

Don't let cooking a whole fish intimidate you! Anyone can make this impressive main course.

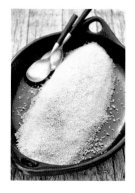

Salt-Crusted Sea Bass with Fennel-Tomato Sauce

3 pounds (1.4 kg) coarse sea salt

1 egg white

1 large (1-pound/ 455-g) whole sea bass, cleaned but with scales left on

a few sprigs thyme and rosemary

1 large fennel bulb

20 cherry tomatoes

toasted sesame oil

1 cup (240 ml) pastis

toasted sesame seeds (see page 135)

Preheat the oven to 350°F (180°C).

In a large bowl, mix the salt with the egg white. Fill the belly of the fish with the thyme and rosemary. Place the fish in a large baking dish (see tip). Cover the fish with the salt mixture and press firmly to adhere. Bake for 20 to 25 minutes.

Meanwhile, thinly slice the fennel and halve the tomatoes.

Heat a large skillet over medium-high heat. Add a splash of sesame oil and the fennel and sauté, stirring. After a few minutes, add the pastis. Simmer for 15 minutes, covered. Add the tomatoes to the skillet and simmer until the fennel is soft, about 5 to 10 minutes.

Pour the fennel and tomato sauce into a pretty bowl, top with the sesame seeds, and place it on the table with the fish in its salt crust. Break the crust open at the table. Now is the fun part (see tip)! Take the entire fish out of the baking dish and place it on a serving platter. Remove the skin (it should come off easily) and serve.

TIP: Baking dish

If you don't have a baking dish large enough to fit the fish, you can also lay it on a rimmed baking sheet. Or, you can cut off the tail to gain some space.

TIP: Removing the fish from the salt crust

Don't be afraid—you'll see how easy this is. Hit the crust with a spoon until it breaks, or insert the spoon along the side of the crust. It will break into large blocks.

Mediterranean Tomato Stew with Calamari

2 or 3 garlic cloves

1 red onion

1 (14-ounce/400-g) can whole peeled tomatoes

2 fresh tomatoes

2 large cleaned squids (1 pound/455 g total)

1 bunch mixed fresh herbs (parsley, dill, rosemary, and so on)

Mince the garlic and cut the onion into rings. Heat a generous splash of olive oil in a saucepan over medium heat. Add the onion and garlic and cook until the onion is translucent. Add the canned tomatoes. Fill the empty can with water and add it to the pan. Simmer for a few minutes.

Meanwhile, cut the fresh tomatoes into cubes. Slice the squid into rings. Add the squid and fresh tomatoes to the tomato sauce. Simmer for 5 minutes, or until the squid is cooked.

Finely chop the herbs and add them to the soup right before serving.

TIP: Rosemary

If you like rosemary, you can cook it in the oil with the garlic from the beginning: This will produce a more pronounced rosemary flavor.

My take on a classic Italian recipe, this warm, fragrant stew is rich with Mediterranean flavor.

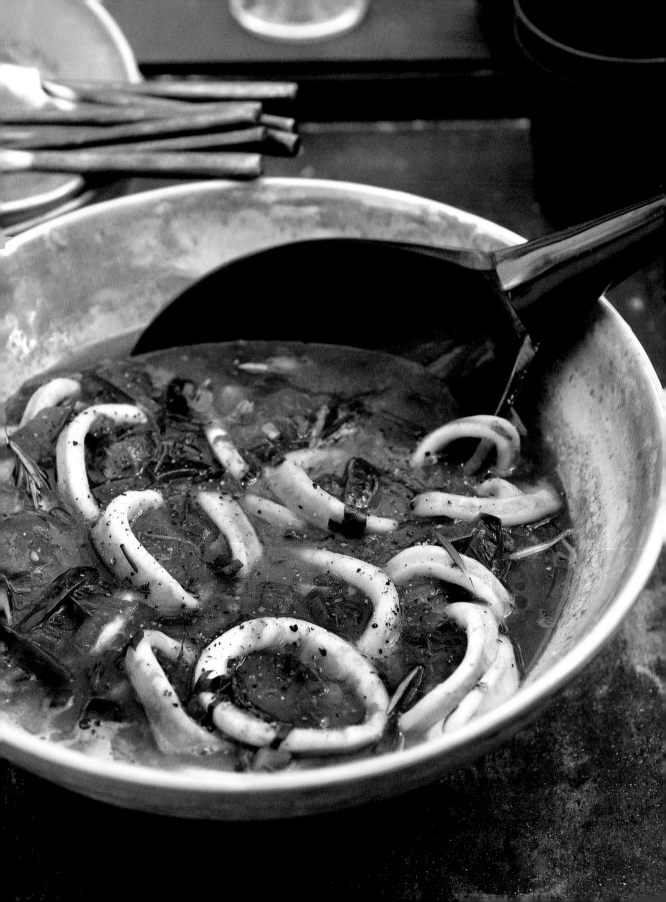

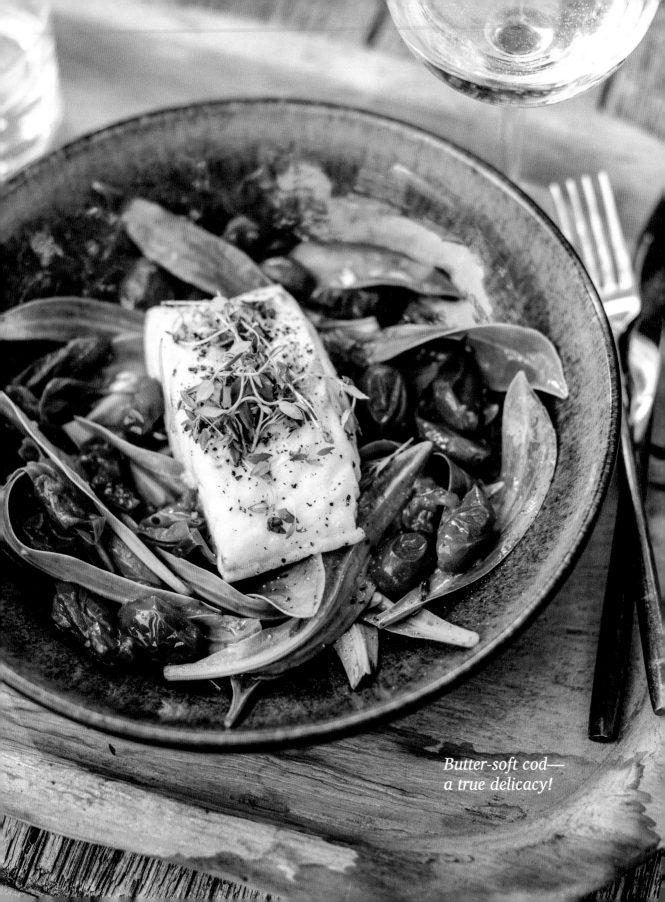

*Butter-soft cod—
a true delicacy!*

Sea Aster Cod with Sautéed Cherry Tomatoes

2 (7-ounce/200-g) cod fillets

30 cherry tomatoes

10½ ounces (300 g) sea aster

fresh thyme

Preheat the oven to 350°F (180°C).

Rub the cod with olive oil; season with pepper and a little salt, and arrange the fish in a baking dish. Bake for 7 to 12 minutes, depending on the thickness of the fillets (see tip).

Halve the cherry tomatoes. Heat a splash of olive oil in a large skillet over medium heat. Add the tomatoes and cook gently until they are soft and release their juices. Season them with pepper and a little salt. Add the sea aster. These leaves should only be warmed; don't let them cook, or they will turn black.

Spoon the tomato mixture onto plates and place the fish on top. Garnish with pepper and thyme.

TIP: Cod cooking time

If the cod is very fresh, just cook it until it has a "glassy" texture—do not let it cook too long, but just until it's no longer raw inside. Toward the end of the cooking time, turn off the oven and leave the cod in for a few more minutes. This will give you butter-soft cod that flakes beautifully.

TIP: Sea aster

Sea aster and samphire (or sea beans; see page 61) are not seaweeds but halophytes—plants that grow in waters with high salinity, like salt marshes. They are rich in iron. Sea aster's fleshy leaves can be eaten raw or cooked, especially the young ones that are softer. They pair well with fish and meat.

Sea aster is also known as "sea spinach." It is a wild perennial plant that grows and spreads itself spontaneously in the wilderness, often found with samphire (sea beans). If you can't find it, you can easily replace it with regular spinach; the dish will still be delicious.

SERVES
2

PREPARATION
10 minutes

COOKING TIME
15 minutes

Lacquered Salmon and Stir-Fried Romano Beans

14 ounces (400 g) Romano beans

3 or 4 garlic cloves

1 (1-inch/2.5-cm) piece fresh ginger

coconut oil

5 to 7 tablespoons (75 to 105 ml) soy sauce

5 to 7 tablespoons (75 to 105 ml) balsamic vinegar

2 (7-ounce/200-g) skin-on salmon fillets

dried thyme

Halve the beans crosswise on a diagonal and thinly slice the garlic and ginger. Heat a generous splash of coconut oil in a skillet over medium-high heat. Add the beans, garlic, and ginger and stir-fry for 5 to 7 minutes.

In a separate skillet, heat the soy sauce and vinegar over high heat. Season the salmon with thyme and a little pepper. Lay the salmon fillets in the bubbling sauce. Cook for 2 minutes on each side, so the salmon is still raw on the inside and the outside is nicely coated with the sauce.

Serve the salmon and beans immediately.

TIP: Stir-fry

For me, stir-frying means cooking while continuously stirring; however, I don't stir-fry at as high a temperature as you traditionally would in certain Asian cuisines. I do this for health reasons: I don't want to burn the ingredients. It is preferable to cook ingredients a little longer at lower heat while stirring continuously.

If you like Japanese cuisine, you will love this wonderful way to prepare salmon with ginger and soy.

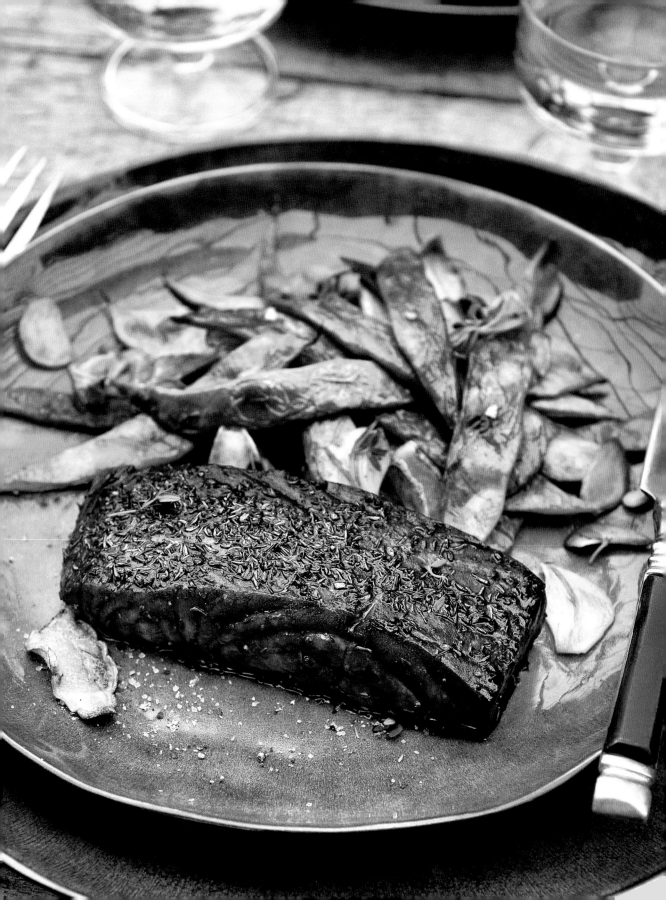

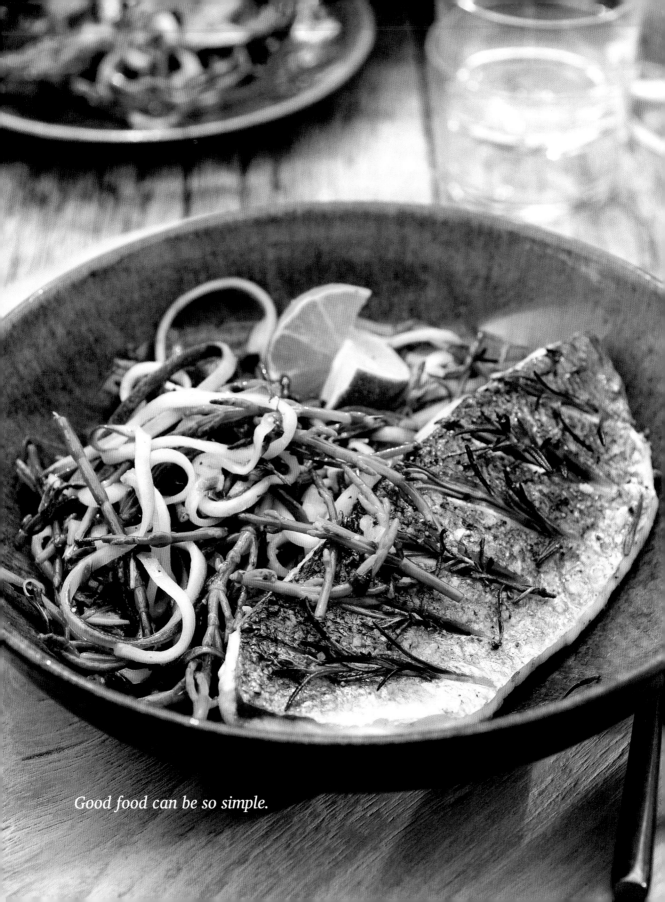

Good food can be so simple.

SERVES
2

PREPARATION
10 minutes

COOKING TIME
15 minutes

Sea Bass with Zucchini and Sea Beans

2 (7-ounce/200-g) skin-on sea bass fillets

1 bunch rosemary, stemmed and chopped

2 large zucchini

7 ounces (200 g) sea beans (also called salicornia or samphire; see tip)

juice of ½ lime

1 bunch basil

Preheat the oven to 350°F (180°C).

Make incisions in the sea bass fillets and fill them with rosemary. Brush the fillets with olive oil. Season with salt and pepper and place the fish in a baking dish. Bake for 15 minutes.

Meanwhile, slice the zucchini lengthwise with a julienne peeler (see tip). Heat a splash of olive oil in a large skillet over medium heat. Add the zucchini and cook for about 2 minutes; the zucchini should remain firm. Add the sea beans and lime juice, and season with pepper. Simmer the mixture for 2 minutes more.

Finely chop the basil. Remove the vegetables from the heat and add the basil.

Arrange the vegetables on plates and place the fish on top.

TIP: Zucchini
Just slice the zucchini until you get to the core where the seeds are. You can use the core for another dish (salad, for instance, or in a soup).

TIP: Sea beans or samphire
Samphire is a bright green sea vegetable with a salty taste. Samphire is often compared to baby asparagus, and its high salt content means that seasoning needn't be added during the cooking process. Quite often, it is simply boiled or steamed with a little olive oil or butter to create a delicious accompaniment to a main meal. It has a strongly oceanic flavor and, therefore, goes wonderfully with seafood.

If samphire is not available, you can use any kind of seaweed, which also has a salty taste.

Red Snapper and Asparagus

4 (3½-ounce/100-g)
red snapper fillets (or
other white-fleshed
fish)

1 bunch asparagus

2 cups (100 g) coarsely
chopped fresh chervil
or parsley

Preheat the oven to 350°F (180°C).

Brush the fish with olive oil; season with salt and pepper and place in a
baking dish. Bake for 15 minutes.

Cut off the hard ends of the asparagus spears. Put the tops in a wide saucepan with a lid; add a little water and a good splash of olive oil. Season with
salt and pepper. Cover the pan and simmer until the asparagus is tender,
6 to 10 minutes.

In a separate saucepan, combine 1 cup (240 ml) water and a splash of olive
oil. Add the chervil and cook until wilted. Season with salt and pepper.
Reserve a small quantity of the chervil for garnish. Puree the rest in a food
processor or blender. Add some water if needed to create a thick soup.

Ladle a little chervil soup into wide, shallow bowls; lay the asparagus in the
middle and garnish with the reserved chervil. Place the fish on top.

TIP: Cooking vegetables
I often cook my vegetables in a small amount of water, with a generous
splash of olive oil, and salt and pepper. This enhances their flavor and
texture.

*The chervil adds an unexpected
nuance to the flavor of this dish—
a delicate hint of anise.*

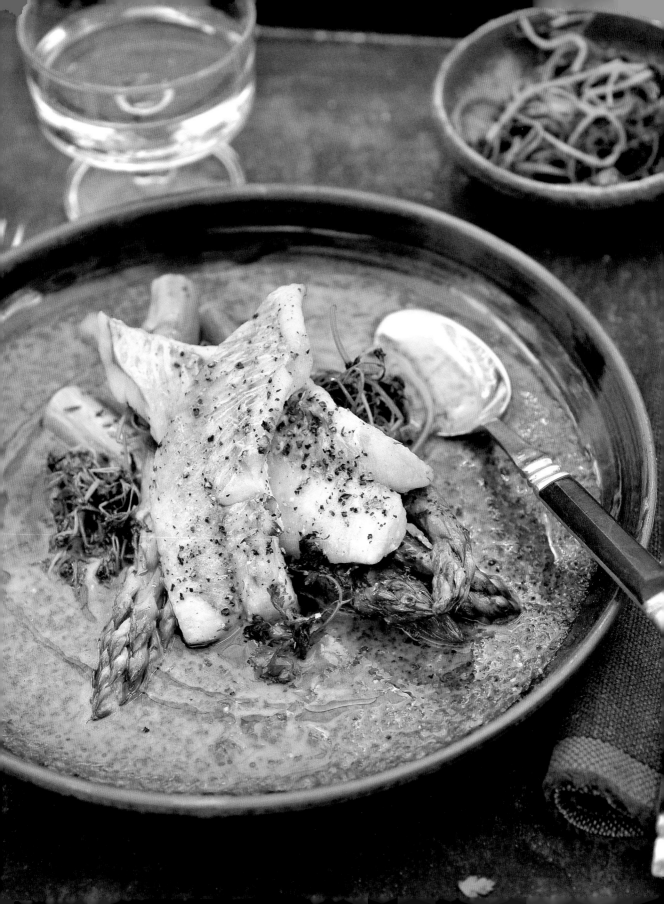

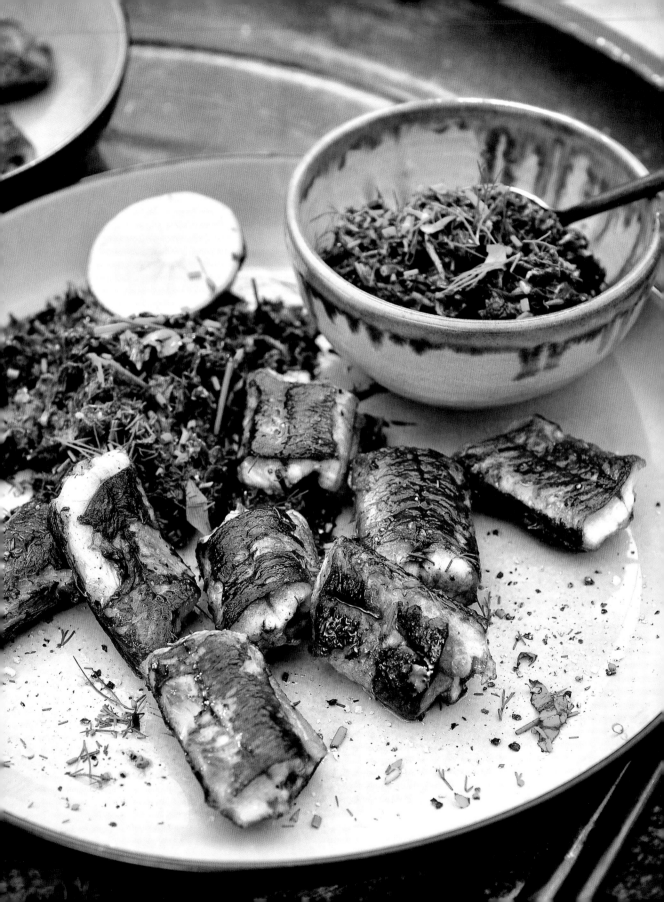

Crispy Fried Eel with Green Herbs

3 eels (about 1 pound/455 g total)

5 ounces (140 g) spinach

1 ounce (20 g) fresh dill

1 ounce (20 g) fresh chives

1 ounce (20 g) fresh parsley

1 ounce (20 g) fresh tarragon

1 ounce (20 g) fresh basil

1 ounce (20 g) fresh cilantro

juice of 1 lime

Cut the eels into 2-inch (5-cm) pieces. Heat a nonstick skillet over medium heat. Add the eel and cook for 15 to 20 minutes, until nicely crisp and swimming in their own fat.

Meanwhile, chop the spinach and herbs very finely. In a separate skillet, heat a splash of olive oil over medium-high heat. Add the spinach and herbs and cook for a few minutes, until the greens are just wilted. Add the lime juice and season with salt and pepper.

Arrange the greens on plates and use a slotted spoon to place the eel alongside. Discard the fat in the pan.

TIP: Fatty fish
Fatty fish such as eel, halibut, and salmon are very healthy and have a high omega-3 content.

TIP: Sorrel/dock
Sorrel is a delicious, sour herb, but is unfortunately very hard to find in stores. Connoisseurs know where they can find it in the wild. I use lime juice to give a sour touch to the greens; however, if you can find sorrel you could certainly add a few leaves to your mix, and you could omit the lime, unless you love the extra-sour touch.

In Belgium and the Netherlands, eel in green sauce is a popular entrée. This is my lighter take on it, but you can easily replace the eel with any other fatty fish, like halibut or salmon. The combination of a fatty fish, cooked until crispy, with the fresh flavor of the herbs, is unforgettable.

SERVES
2

PREPARATION
15 minutes

COOKING TIME
15 to 20 minutes

Salmon with Olive-Pistachio Tapenade and Tomatoes

½ cup (100 g) green olives, pitted

generous ⅓ cup (50 g) shelled pistachios

2 (7-ounce/200-g) salmon fillets

10 ounces (280 g) cherry tomatoes with stems

dried thyme

a few sprigs dill, chopped

Preheat the oven to 350°F (180°C).

Finely chop the olives and pistachios and transfer them to a small bowl. Add a splash of olive oil and stir to combine.

Put the fish in a baking dish. Spread the olive mixture around and between the fillets.

Put the tomatoes in a separate baking dish. Season with salt, pepper, and thyme, and sprinkle with olive oil. Bake the fish and tomatoes for 15 minutes until the fish is opaque in center.

Top with a little dill and serve.

This dish is even more beautiful if you make it for guests, as shown here. Just double or triple the recipe. You can prepare everything in advance and when people arrive you just have to put it in the oven.

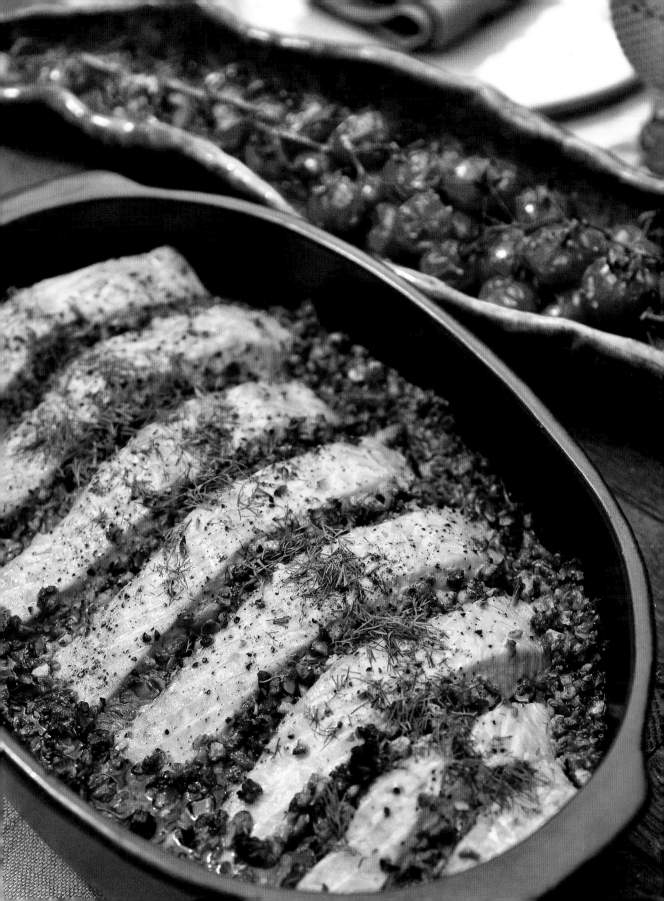

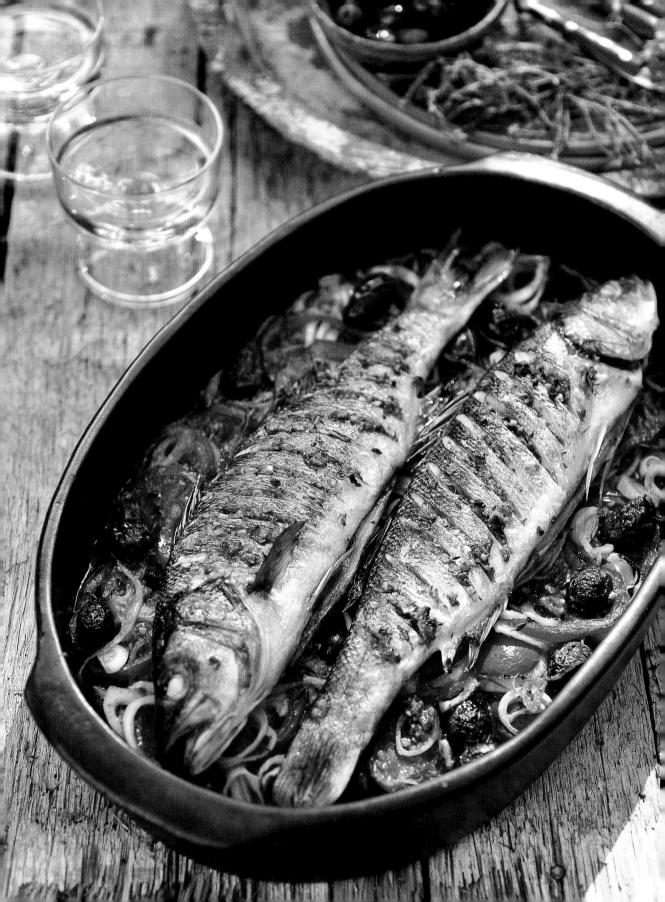

Sea Bass with Anchovies, Tomatoes, and Onions

6 tomatoes

3 medium yellow onions

handful of olives (see tip)

12 anchovy fillets

4 garlic cloves

1 teaspoon dried thyme

2 (9- to 11-ounce/255- to 310-g) skin-on, whole sea bass

Core and thinly slice the tomatoes; thinly slice the onions. Transfer them to a baking dish and add the olives, a splash of olive oil, salt, and pepper. Stir to combine.

Finely chop the anchovy fillets and the garlic. In a bowl, mix the anchovies and garlic with the thyme. Season with pepper and a splash of olive oil (do not add salt, because the anchovies are salty).

Rinse the fish and make a deep incision (cutting to the bone) every ½ inch (12 mm) on the body on both sides. Fill the incisions with the anchovy mixture. Lay the sea bass over the vegetables in the baking dish and bake for 15 to 20 minutes until the thickest part of the fish flakes easily. Serve the fish straight from the baking dish, as shown.

TIP: Olives
You can choose any olives you like, including marinated olives. Taste them first: If you like them cold, you will also like them cooked.

The anchovies add a natural salty flavor and make all the difference!

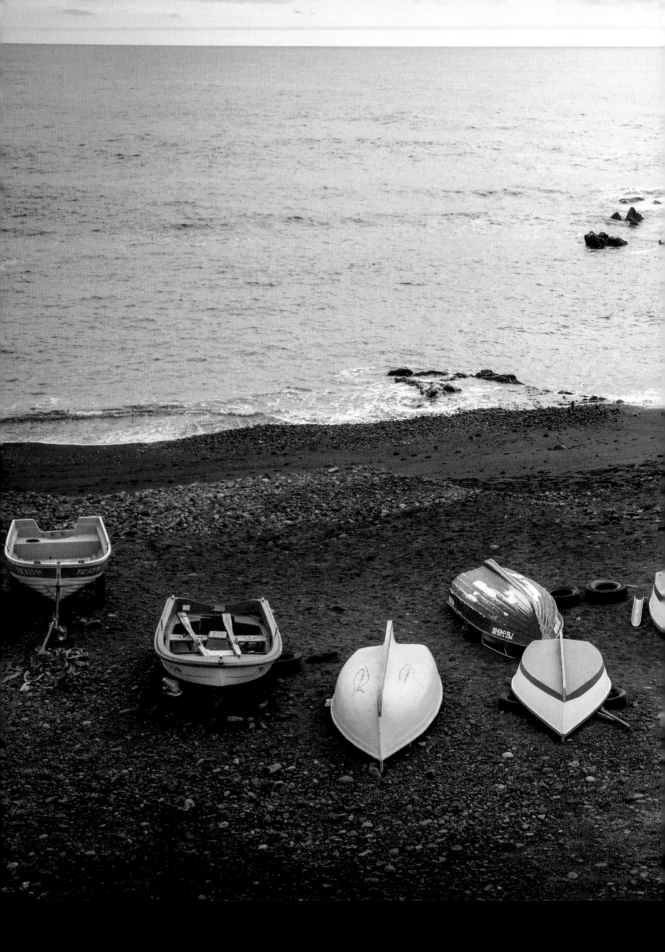

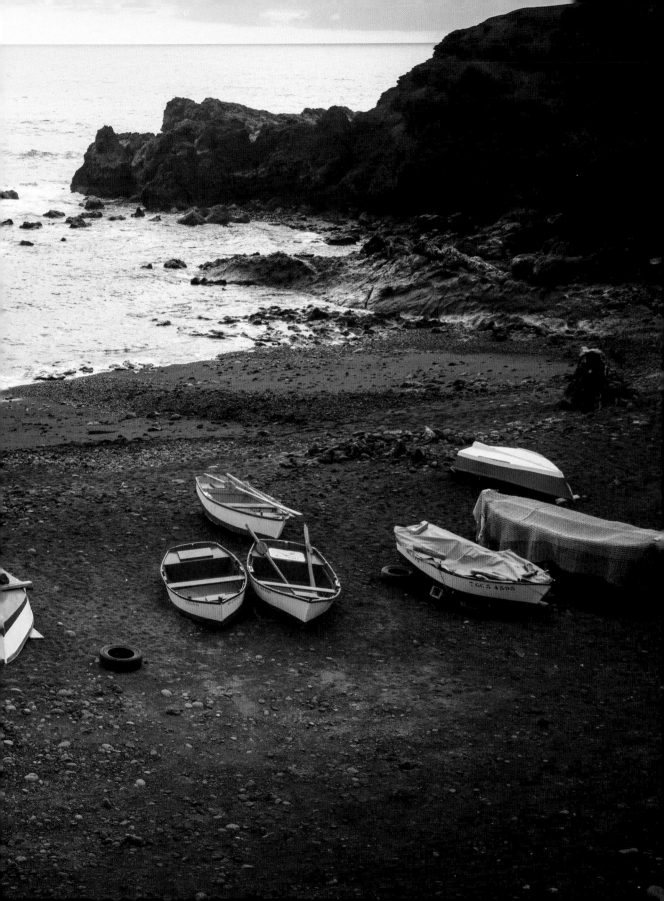

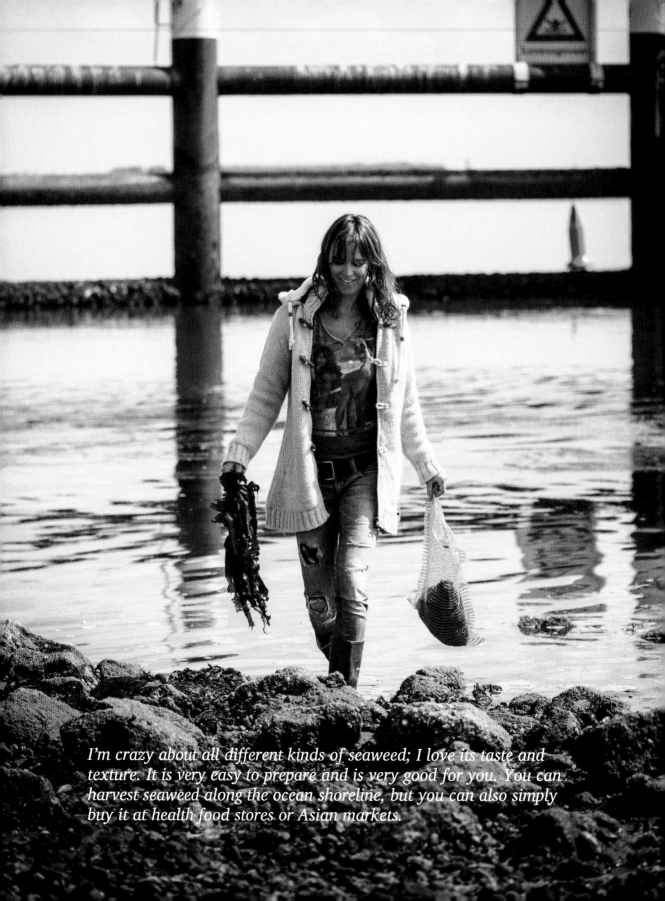

I'm crazy about all different kinds of seaweed; I love its taste and texture. It is very easy to prepare and is very good for you. You can harvest seaweed along the ocean shoreline, but you can also simply buy it at health food stores or Asian markets.

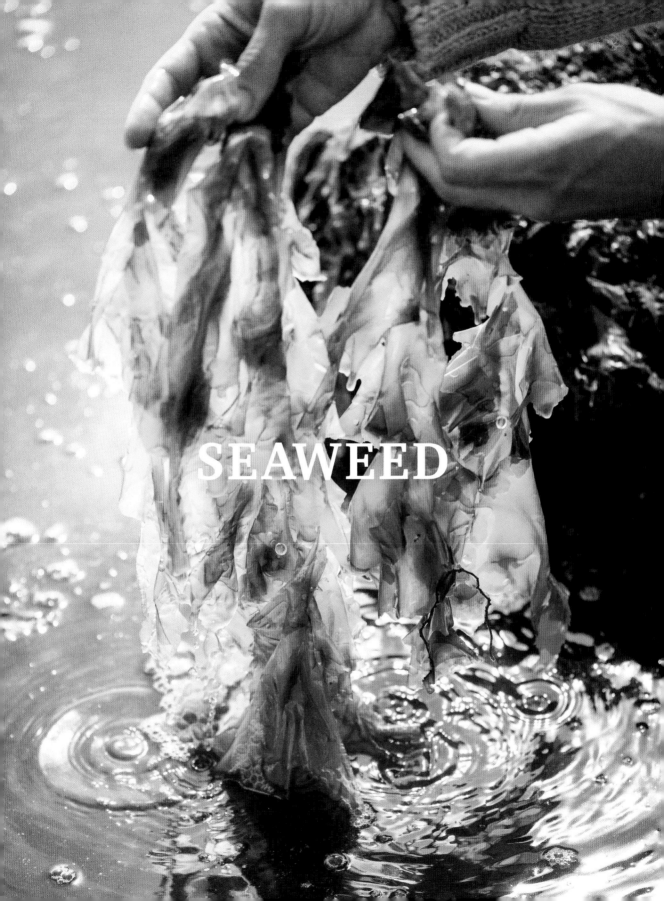

SEAWEED

MAKES
40 to 50 chips

PREPARATION
5 minutes

COOKING TIME
3 to 5 minutes

Nori Chips

10 nori sheets (see tip)

fleur de sel

Preheat the oven to 350°F (180°C).

Fill a small bowl with water and a separate small bowl with olive oil.

Brush one side of each nori sheet with olive oil and season with a little fleur de sel. Fold the sheets in two with the oiled sides together. Brush water on both outer sides. This will soften the nori sheet.

Cut the sheets into the desired chip shapes. I always make them into triangles— easy and simple. Place the triangles on a baking sheet. Bake for 3 to 5 minutes, until crispy. Stay nearby and check them regularly so that they do not burn.

TIP: Nori

Nori is one of the best known kinds of seaweed. But I strongly recommend you experiment with other seaweeds, such as arame, dulse, hijiki, and wakame. Seaweed has been eaten and enjoyed for a long time all over the world. Of all the plants on earth, they are the ones with the most minerals, including iodine, iron, magnesium, and potassium. Most of them are also a good source of calcium (calcium is not exclusively found in dairy products), and vitamins A, B_6, C, and E. Seaweed is also easy to digest because aquatic plants have a soft texture.

You can find nori sheets in many grocery stores, and other types of seaweeds can be found in health food stores and Asian markets. They are usually sold dry, which is convenient because dried seaweed has a long shelf life.

Dried seaweeds are also very easy to prepare. First soak them in water until rehydrated, and then cook them with vegetables, lentils, chickpeas, or fish. Simple, tasty, and healthy.

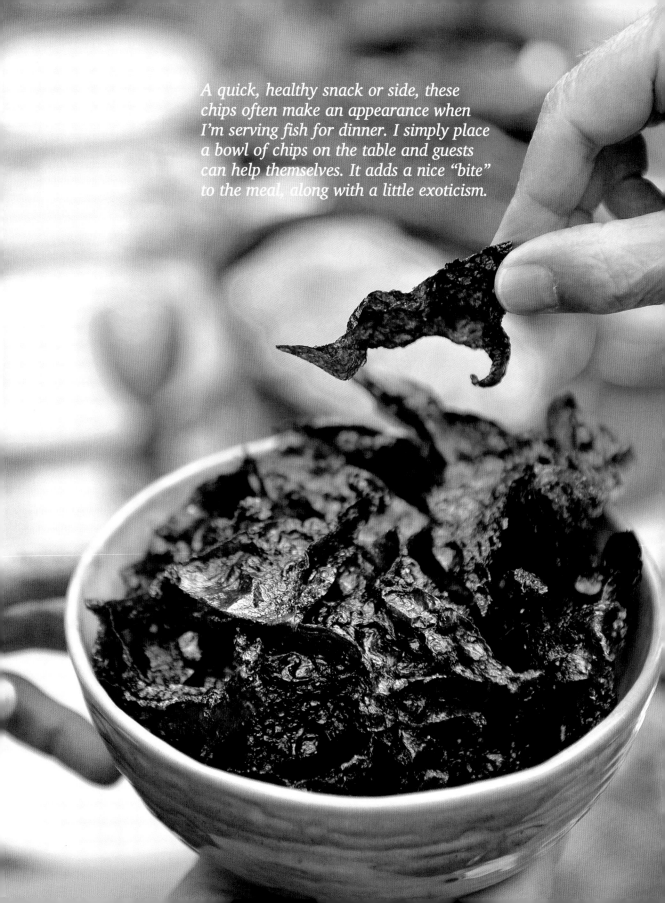

A quick, healthy snack or side, these chips often make an appearance when I'm serving fish for dinner. I simply place a bowl of chips on the table and guests can help themselves. It adds a nice "bite" to the meal, along with a little exoticism.

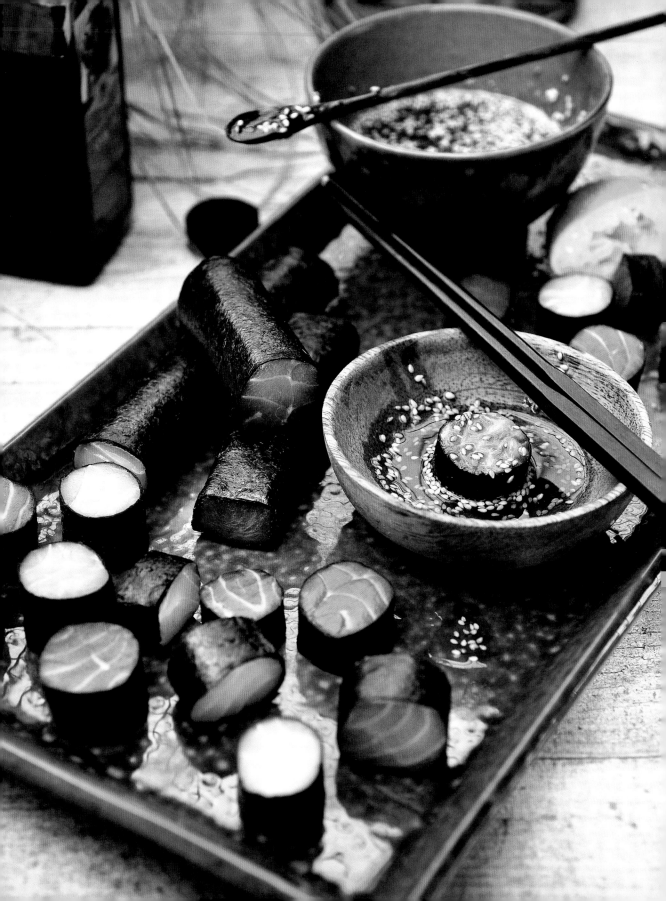

Sashimi Rolls

7 ounces (200 g) fish fillet of your choice (see tip)

5 nori sheets

¼ cup (60 ml) soy sauce

1 teaspoon toasted sesame seeds (see page 135)

lime wedges

Slice the fish into five long, thick strips. Brush the nori sheets with water; lay them flat on your work surface and roll a fish strip in each of them. Let sit for a few minutes. Cut the rolls crosswise into small pieces.

In a small bowl, mix the soy sauce, 2 tablespoons olive oil, and the sesame seeds.

Serve the sashimi with the sauce and lime wedges.

TIP: Which fish?

Choose firm, thick, boneless fillets with the skin removed. I have a preference for salmon, albacore tuna, and sea bass. Cod works too, although it doesn't have a lot of flavor. No matter which kind you select, just make sure it is very fresh. I always ask my fishmonger if the fish is sashimi quality.

You could see this preparation as a mix between sushi and sashimi. Taste it, and you will not miss the rice. This combination is perfect just as it is: fish, seaweed, soy sauce, and toasted sesame seeds.

MAKES
8 to 10 wraps

PREPARATION
20 minutes

COOKING TIME
20 minutes

Fish Wraps with Sesame-Soy Dipping Sauce

¼ ounce (7 g) arame seaweed (optional, see tip)

3 leeks (see tip)

1⅓ cups (40 g) coarsely chopped fresh herbs (cilantro, parsley, chives, and so on)

fleur de sel

10½ ounces (300 g) firm-fleshed fish (such as salmon, cod, or similar), cut into 8 to 10 pieces

5 nori sheets, cut in half with scissors

For the dipping sauce:

3 tablespoons soy sauce

2 tablespoons toasted sesame seeds (see page 135)

1 lime (½ for juice and ½ for wedges)

Preheat the oven to 350°F (180°C).

Soak the arame in water for 5 minutes, if using.

Remove and discard the tough outer layers of the leeks and cut the leeks into 4-inch (10-cm) pieces. Rinse them well to remove any grit between the leaves. Place the leeks in a saucepan and add water to cover and a little olive oil. Drain the arame, if using, and add it to the pan with the leeks. Bring to a simmer over medium-high heat and cook for 15 minutes.

Place the herbs in a bowl, add a splash of olive oil, and season with fleur de sel and pepper.

Brush a nori sheet with water, put some fresh herbs in the center, and top with a piece of the fish. Wrap the nori around the fish and herbs. If necessary, brush the ends with water so you can seal the nori. Place the wraps in a baking dish. Bake for 15 minutes.

Meanwhile, make the dipping sauce: In a small bowl stir together ¼ cup (60 ml) olive oil, the soy sauce, sesame seeds, and lime juice.

Drain the leeks and arame. Arrange them on a serving platter and sprinkle with a little of the dipping sauce. Add the nori wraps and serve with lime wedges and the dipping sauce.

TIP: Arame

Arame seaweed is an ideal seaweed for beginners: The taste is rather sweet and nutty. Popular in Asian cuisine, it has found its way into many natural foods stores in the West and is appreciated for its health benefits. Arame has lots of iodine, calcium, fiber, and minerals. With soaking and cooking, arame expands up to five times its original volume.

TIP: Leeks

In the spring, you can sometimes find young leeks, and there is no need to remove their outer layers. If you use winter leeks, you should remove the three outer layers because they remain tough (even after cooking) and cut the inner layers into small pieces.

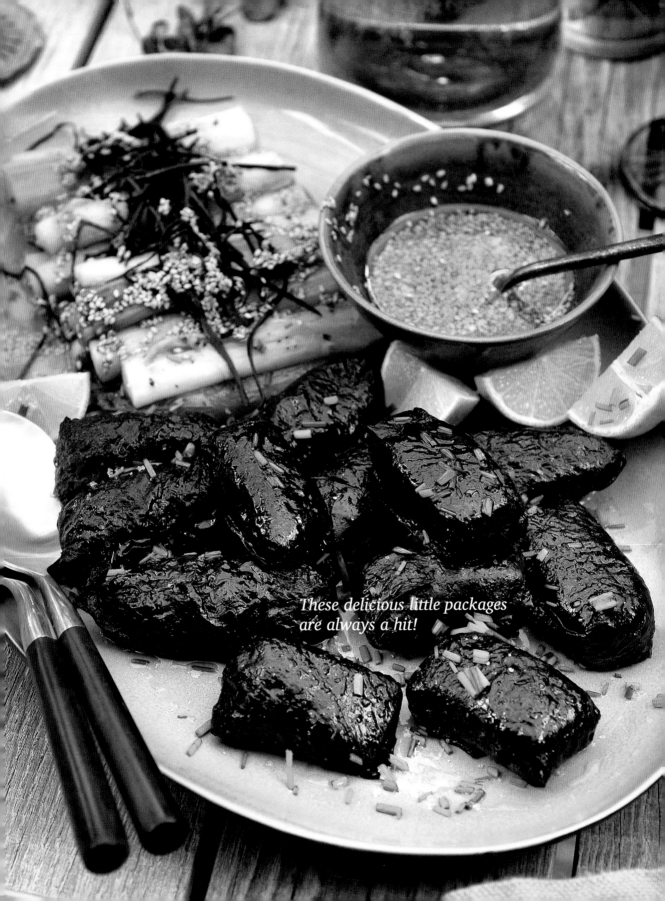

These delicious little packages
are always a hit!

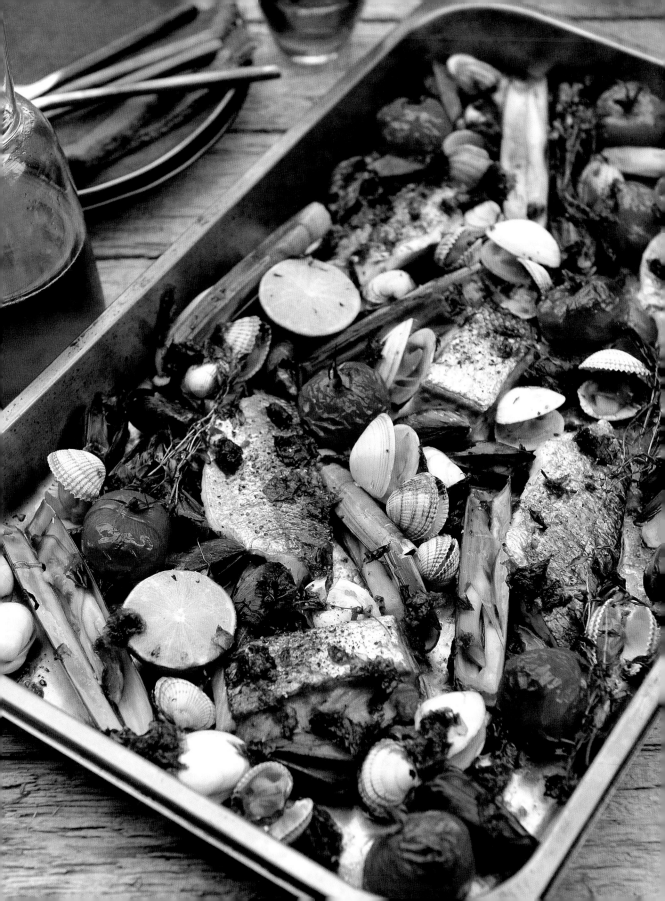

Fish and Shellfish Roasted with Tomatoes and Sea Lettuce

10 mussels

10 cockles

4 razor clams

10½ ounces (300 g) skin-on fish fillets (salmon, sea bass, and gilt-head bream are good choices)

8 to 10 small tomatoes

1 lime, halved

1¾ ounces (50 g) fresh seaweed (see tip)

a few sprigs thyme

Preheat the oven to 350°F (180°C).

Scrub the mussels, cockles, and clams.

Coat a large baking dish with olive oil and sprinkle with salt and pepper. Arrange the fish fillets, skin side up, in the baking dish. Arrange the tomatoes, lime halves, and mussels around the fish. Sprinkle with olive oil and season with salt and pepper. Bake for 7 minutes.

Meanwhile, rinse the seaweed, squeeze out the water, and place in a bowl. Spread the seaweed branches and add a little olive oil. Season with a little salt and pepper. Rub the thyme sprigs with oil.

After 7 minutes, remove the baking dish from the oven, add the cockles and clams, and sprinkle the seaweed and thyme over the entire dish. Return to the oven and bake for 10 minutes more. Discard any shellfish that do not open. Serve immediately.

TIP: Fresh seaweed

You can purchase fresh seaweed at good supermarkets. I used sea lettuce here, but any kind could work. If you can't find fresh seaweed, tear nori seaweed into strips and mix with a little olive oil. Sprinkle the nori pieces over the dish 3 to 5 minutes before the cooking time is done.

This rustic, colorful, and romantic meal is meant to be shared with people you love. Just place the baking dish on the table and let everyone help themselves.

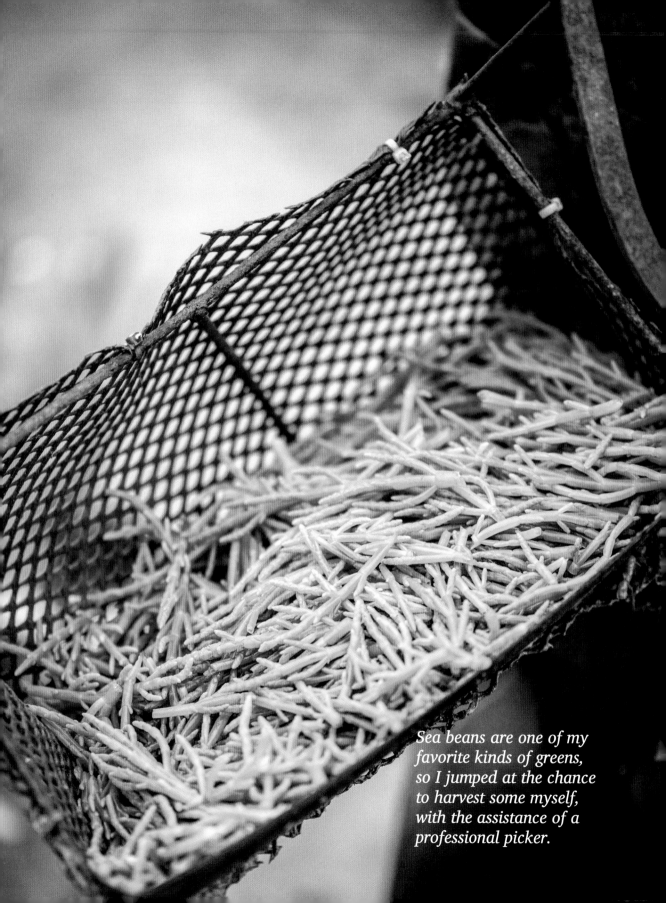

Sea beans are one of my favorite kinds of greens, so I jumped at the chance to harvest some myself, with the assistance of a professional picker.

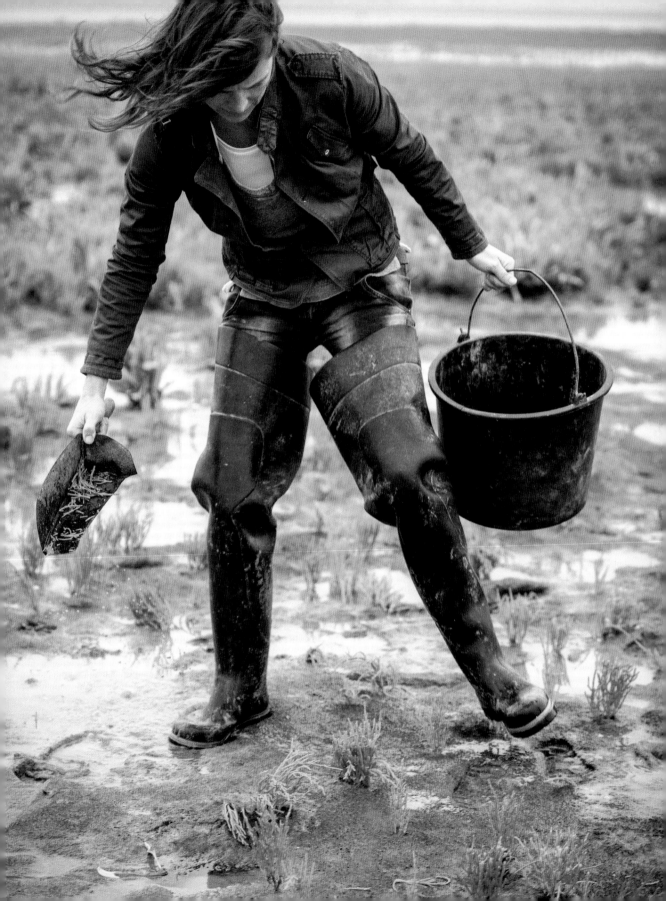

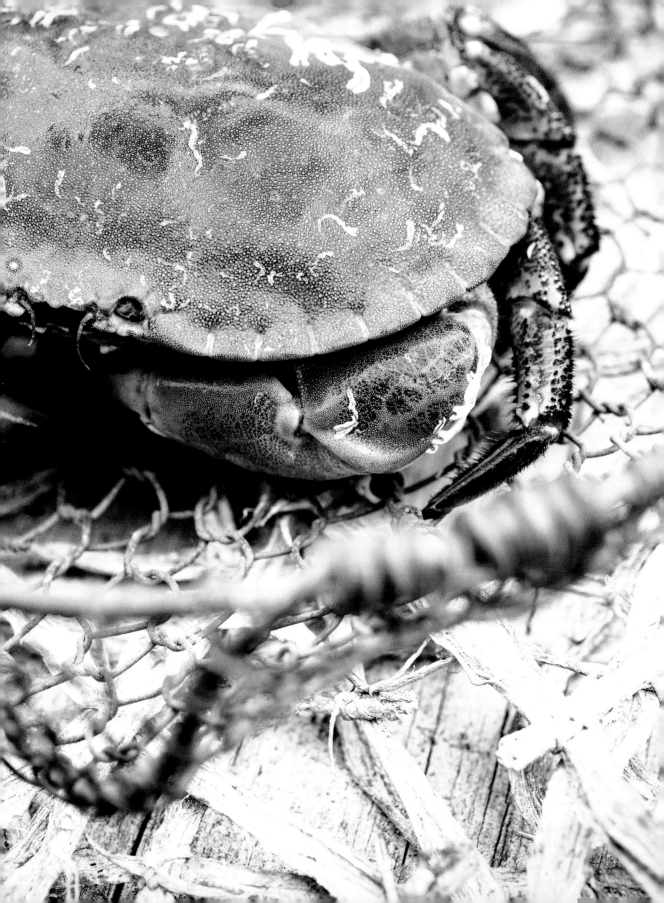

SHELLFISH

Crabs Stuffed with Tomatoes, Basil, and Hazelnuts

2 fresh 1 to 1½-pound (455- to 680-g) Dungeness crabs, or 10½ ounces (300 g) canned crabmeat or fresh lump crabmeat

5 ounces (140 g) peeled cooked shrimp (see tip)

1 bunch basil

2 scallions

2 tomatoes

handful of toasted hazelnuts

hazelnut oil

fleur de sel

Pull the crab legs from the body with a twist. Be careful not to break the shell. Remove the meat from the legs and body. (This is a messy job that takes time. However, read the last tip—it will give you courage.) Put the crabmeat in a bowl, reserving a few of the nicest pieces. Clean the crab shells well.

Chop the shrimp. Chop the basil and scallions. Core, seed, and chop the tomatoes. Coarsely chop the hazelnuts. Add the tomatoes, hazelnuts, and shrimp to the bowl with the crabmeat. Sprinkle with a splash of hazelnut oil and season with pepper and a little fleur de sel. Mix carefully.

Fill the shells with this mixture. Set the nicest pieces of crabmeat on top and serve.

TIP: Roe
In addition to the white crabmeat, females contain roe, also known as red coral. Not everyone is wild about the roe, but it is actually delicious, if a bit rich. You can add this to the crab mixture, or you could serve it on the side by mixing it with mayonnaise to create a dressing.

TIP: Shrimp
You will never get enough meat from a crab to completely fill the shell; therefore, I fill it out with shrimp. This way, you won't have to worry about having a generously filled crab.

TIP: 1 hour or 15 minutes?
Removing crabmeat is a lot of work. After a meal, I clean the crab shells so I can reuse them. Then, for a quick meal, I make the filling with canned crabmeat or fresh lump crabmeat and the entire dish is ready in 15 minutes.

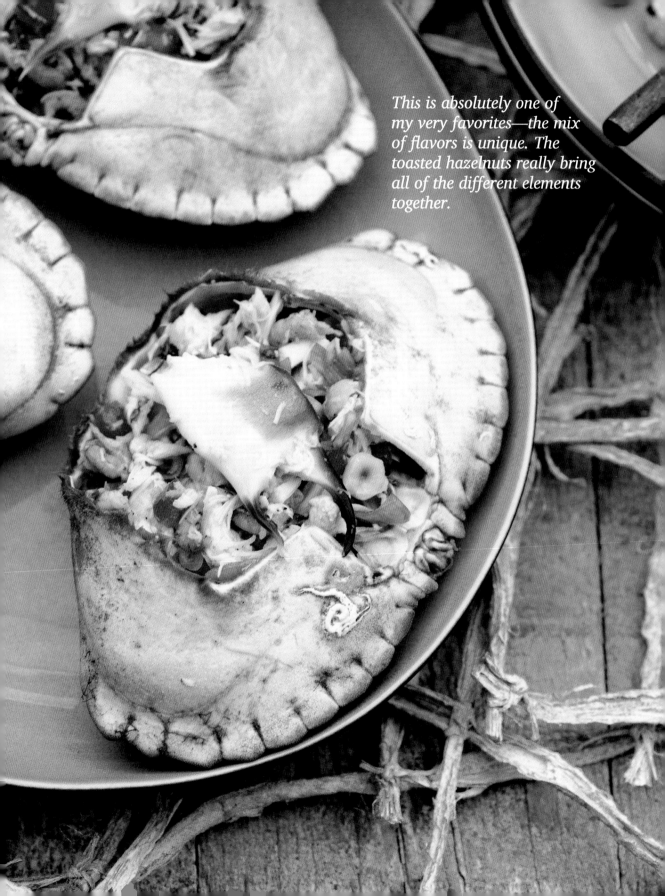

This is absolutely one of my very favorites—the mix of flavors is unique. The toasted hazelnuts really bring all of the different elements together.

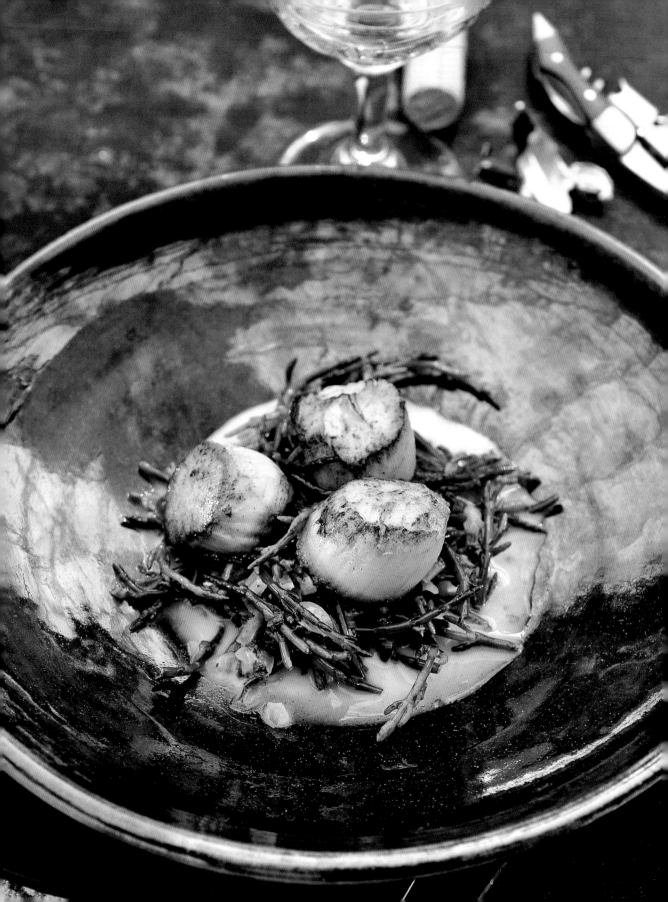

Seared Scallops with Sea Beans

1 shallot

3 to 4 tablespoons (30 to 55 g) good-quality butter

handful of curly parsley

1 cup (240 ml) white wine

juice of 1 lime

3½ ounces (100 g) sea beans (also called salicornia or samphire, see page 61)

6 sea scallops

Mince the shallot. Melt half the butter in a small skillet. Add the shallot.

Meanwhile, finely chop the parsley. When the shallot is translucent, add the wine and parsley. Simmer for a few minutes, then add the lime juice.

In a separate skillet, briefly heat the sea beans in some olive oil over medium heat (see tip).

In a third skillet, melt the remaining butter. Add the scallops and sear for 2 minutes on each side. Season with salt and pepper.

Spoon the parsley sauce into soup plates, arrange the sea beans over the sauce, set the scallops on top, and serve.

TIP: Sea beans

Sea beans don't need cooking—they should only be warmed. They become darker, less attractive, and less flavorful the longer they cook. In addition, sea beans do not need a lot of seasoning, as they are naturally salty.

Try serving this as a first course. The shallot, butter, and parsley sauce is the perfect complement to the sea beans and the scallops.

SERVES
5 to 8 as an appetizer

PREPARATION
15 minutes

COOKING TIME
15 minutes

Wonderful Shrimp Fritters

9 ounces (255 g) medium or jumbo peeled shrimp

2 garlic cloves

1 (½-inch/12-mm) piece fresh ginger

¼ cup (10 g) coarsely chopped fresh basil

2 scallions

2 tablespoons red curry paste

1 egg white

outer leaves of red cabbage, trimmed (see tip)

Peel the shrimp, deveining them, if necessary, and very finely chop them. Mince the garlic. Peel and mince the ginger. Thinly slice the basil and scallions.

In a bowl, combine the garlic, ginger, basil, scallions, and curry paste. Lightly whisk in the egg white.

Stir the shrimp into the curry paste mixture.

Heat a few tablespoons of olive oil or coconut oil in a large skillet over medium-high heat. Use a tablespoon to drop mounds of the shrimp mixture (which should be somewhat liquid) into the oil and fry, turning once, until the fritters are lightly browned and the shrimp is cooked through (if you cut into a fritter, any visible shrimp should be pink). Using a slotted spoon, transfer the fritters to a paper towel–lined plate to drain. Repeat until you have used all the shrimp mixture, adding more oil as needed.

Arrange the cabbage leaves on a serving plate. Spear the fritters with toothpicks, place them on the cabbage leaves, and serve.

TIP: Red cabbage
The outer leaves of red cabbage have an unbelievably pretty color—somewhere between green, purple, and wine-red. Unfortunately, in many supermarkets, the outer leaves of red cabbage are removed before they arrive on the shelves. Your local farmers' market is a good place to look for whole cabbages. Select the most vibrantly colored leaves and trim them into circles, just larger than the fritters.

A great appetizer to serve when you have guests, these fritters are so tasty and they look gorgeous against the colorful cabbage leaves.

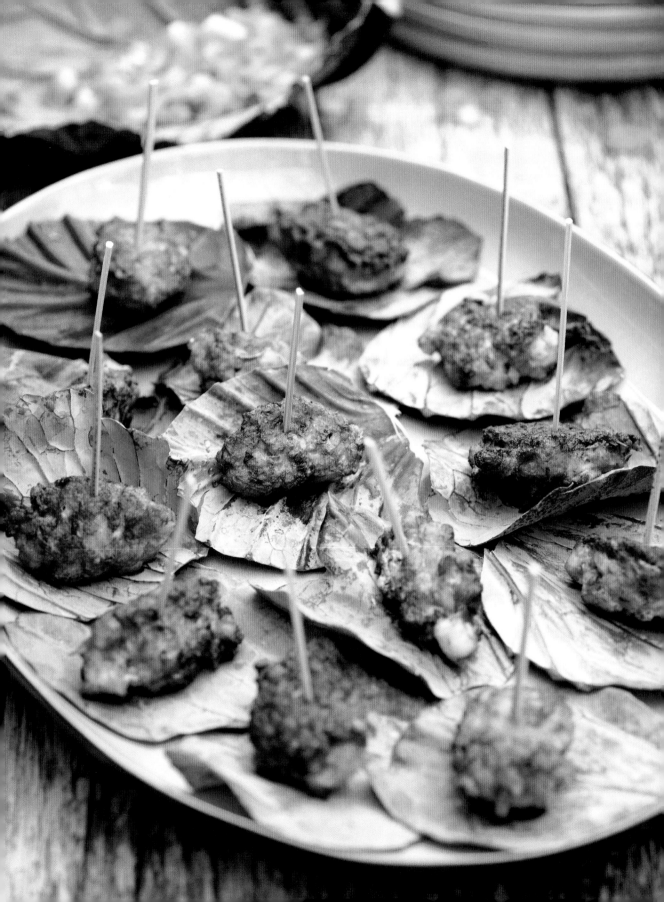

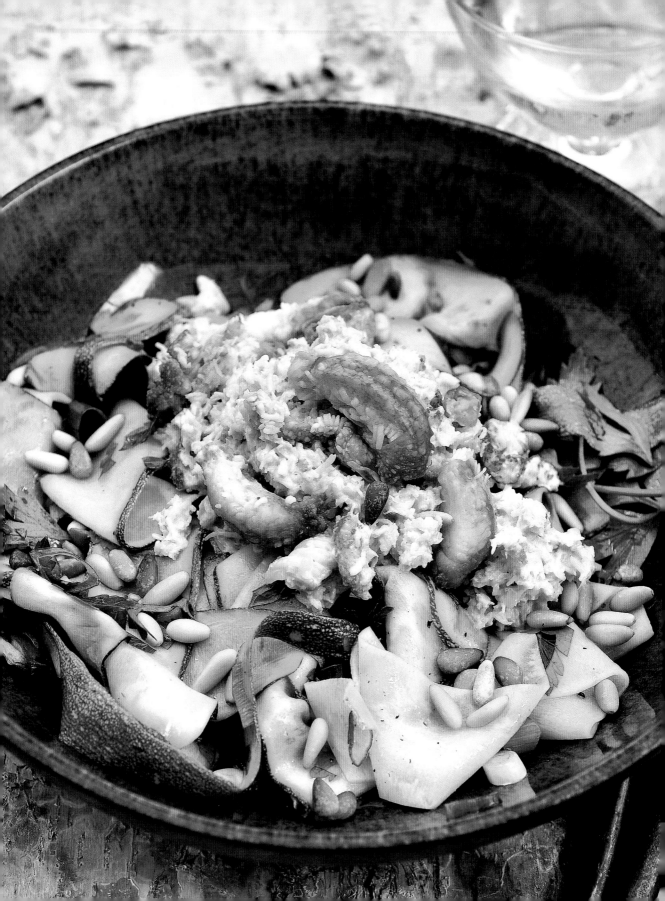

Zucchini Noodles with Crab

1 large zucchini

handful of pine nuts

2 scallions

1 bunch flat-leaf parsley

7 ounces (200 g) fresh lump or canned crabmeat

2 tablespoons mayonnaise (see tip)

Preheat the oven to 350°F (180°C).

Use a vegetable peeler to slice the zucchini lengthwise into long, noodlelike strips. Arrange the noodles in a baking dish, season with salt and pepper, and sprinkle with olive oil. Lightly toss and bake for 10 to 15 minutes, until the noodles are evenly softened.

Spread the pine nuts on a small baking sheet and toast in the oven for 7 minutes, or until they begin to brown.

Meanwhile, chop the scallions and parsley. Drain the crabmeat and combine it with the mayonnaise in a small bowl.

Combine the zucchini, scallions, and parsley in a serving bowl. Arrange the crabmeat on top and finish with the toasted pine nuts.

TIP: Zucchini
Just slice zucchini until you get to the core where the seeds are. You can use the core for another dish (salad, for instance, or in a soup).

TIP: Homemade mayonnaise
Making it at home is so simple and so tasty! Try it once and you'll never want to eat store-bought again. See page 97 for instructions on how to make it.

For me, this is the perfect meal—tasty, easy to make, unique, and healthy. The tender zucchini goes well with the crabmeat. The mayonnaise binds all of the flavors together, and the toasted pine nuts provide a crispy touch.

Cockles with Leeks and Sugar Snap Peas

2 pounds (910 g) cockles (see tip)

1 leek

3½ ounces (100 g) sugar snap peas

toasted sesame oil

2 garlic cloves

1 (1½-inch/4-cm) piece fresh ginger

juice of 1 lemon

1 cup (240 ml) white wine

3 tablespoons soy sauce

3 scallions

1⅓ cups (40 g) coarsely chopped fresh cilantro

toasted sesame seeds (see page 135)

Rinse the cockles several times in cold water.

Slice the leek crosswise into rings and rinse well in a colander to remove any grit. Combine the leeks, peas, and a splash of toasted sesame oil in a saucepan and set over medium-high heat. Mince the garlic, peel and grate the ginger, and add both to the pan along with the lemon juice. Simmer, stirring frequently, until the leek is soft. Add the wine and soy sauce, then place the cockles on top. Cover the pan and simmer for 7 minutes, or until all the cockles open; discard any that do not open.

Meanwhile, finely chop the scallions and cilantro.

Remove the pot from the heat and add the scallions and cilantro.

Spoon the cockles and vegetables into bowls and garnish with toasted sesame seeds.

TIP: Cockles
I love cockles; my father always used to buy them from local fishermen. Cockles are very seasonal, and they are smaller than most other shellfish, which is why they are so cute. If I can't find cockles, I use mussels or clams.

Normally, shellfish are prepared with few or no vegetables, which is really a pity. Just try this recipe and you will see that cockles, mussels, or clams combine perfectly with leeks and sugar snap peas.

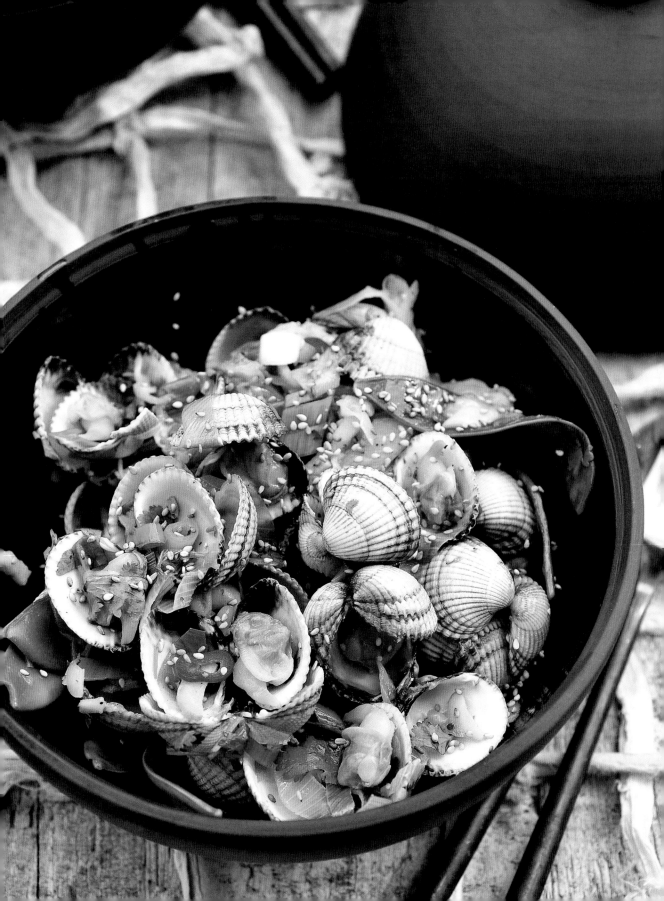

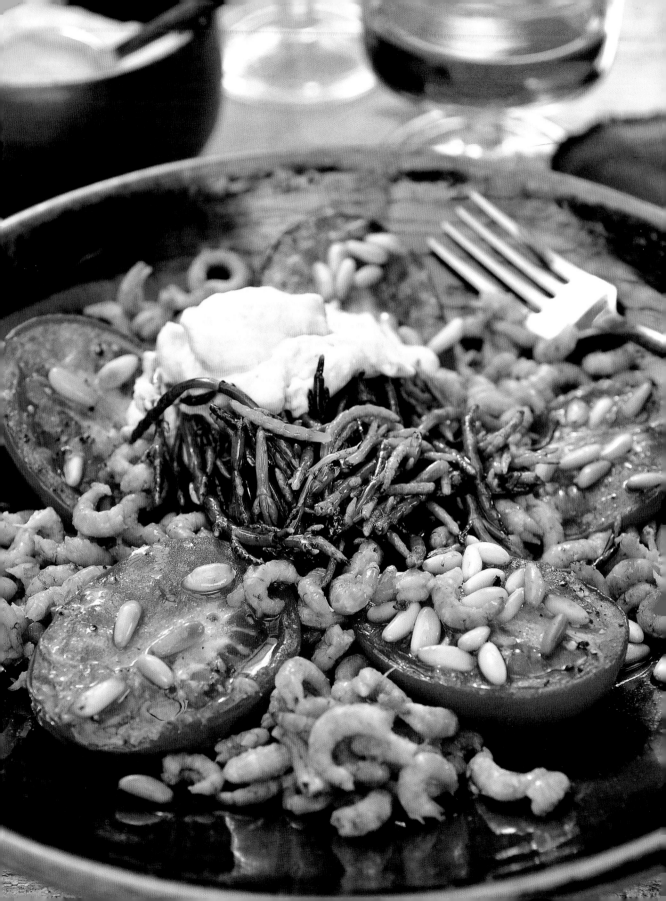

Shrimp-Topped Roasted Tomatoes

SERVES
2

PREPARATION
15 minutes

COOKING TIME
15 minutes

4 or 5 tomatoes (preferably Roma tomatoes)

handful of pine nuts

For the mayonnaise:

2 egg yolks

smooth mustard (like Dijon)

juice of 1 lemon (or to taste)

7 ounces (200 g) sea beans (also called salicornia or samphire, see page 61)

juice of 1 lemon

10 ounces (280 g) peeled cooked shrimp (see tip)

Preheat the oven to 350°F (180°C).

Core and halve the tomatoes; place them in a baking dish, cut side up. Sprinkle with olive oil and season with salt and pepper. Add the pine nuts and bake for 15 minutes.

Meanwhile, make the mayonnaise: Put the egg yolks in a blender. Add 1 tablespoon mustard and 1 tablespoon extra-virgin olive oil. Blend briefly. With the motor running, slowly add more oil in a steady stream. Stop when you have the desired quantity and consistency. Add lemon juice, additional mustard, salt, and pepper to taste. If you find your mayonnaise is too thick, add a little water. (It is important to add mustard in the beginning, since it is the primary binding agent, but then you can add more later to achieve your desired flavor.)

Heat a little olive oil in a skillet over medium-high heat. Add the sea beans and lemon juice and season with pepper. Cook just until the sea beans are warmed through.

Put the cooked tomatoes in a circle on the edge of a serving plate and the sea beans in the middle, and sprinkle the shrimp and pine nuts over the tomatoes. Dollop some mayonnaise on top of the sea beans and serve.

TIP: Shrimp

I use North Sea shrimp, which are tiny shrimp common in Belgium and the Netherlands. They do not stay fresh for long, so they are cooked right on the fishing boats as soon as they're hauled in. However, for this dish, you can use any other cooked shrimp, even large ones.

This dish is an unexpected combination of hot and cold—the warm roasted tomatoes and the cool mayonnaise and shrimp. It sits comfortably between salad starter and main course. I love it!

SERVES
2

PREPARATION
15 minutes

COOKING TIME
30 minutes

Divine Fish Stew

1 red bell pepper

3 garlic cloves

2 (14-ounce/400-g) cans whole peeled tomatoes

1 cup (240 ml) red wine

5 ounces (140 g) salmon fillet

5 ounces (140 g) firm white-fleshed fish fillet

7 ounces (198 g) mussels

6 large shrimp

1 bunch flat-leaf parsley

Seed and dice the bell pepper. Mince the garlic. Pour a generous glug of olive oil into a large deep pot, add the garlic and bell pepper, and cook over medium-high heat until soft. Add the tomatoes, wine, and 1 cup (240 ml) water. Cover and cook for about 15 minutes.

Meanwhile, cut the fish into large pieces; rinse the mussels, and peel and devein the shrimp, leaving the tails on. Add the fish, shrimp, and mussels to the soup; cover and simmer for 10 minutes more. Check for mussels that have not opened and discard them.

Chop the parsley and sprinkle it over the soup, then serve.

The red wine gives this sophisticated soup a deep red color and a warm, complex flavor.

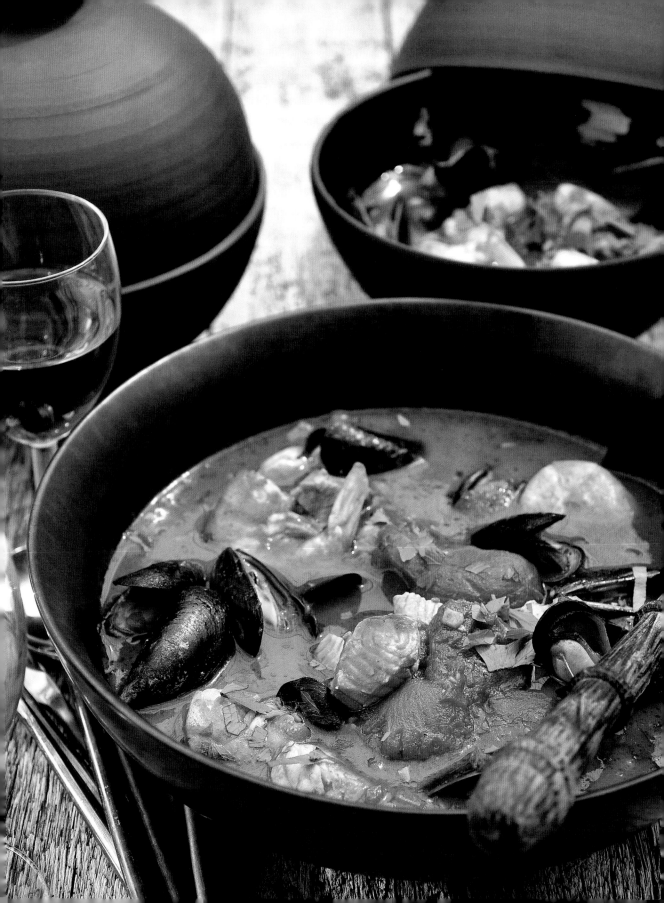

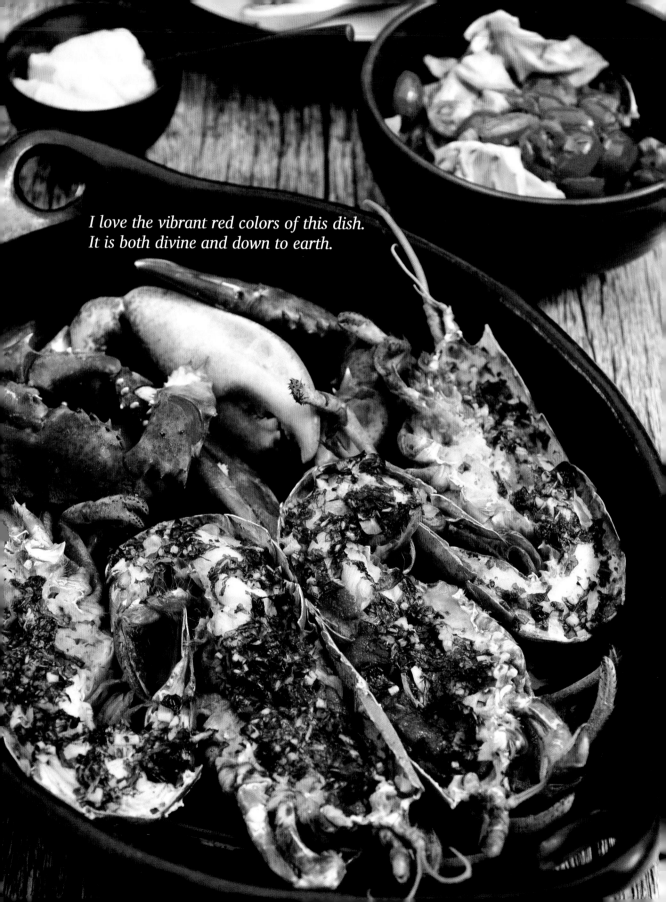

I love the vibrant red colors of this dish.
It is both divine and down to earth.

Baked Lobster with Warm Tomato Salad

1 pint (10 ounces/ 280 g) cherry tomatoes

2 live lobsters (about 1⅓ pounds/600 g each)

1⅓ cups (40 g) coarsely chopped fresh basil

1 garlic clove

juice of 1 lime

7 ounces (200 g) butter lettuce

1 bunch chives

2 tablespoons mayonnaise (preferably homemade; see page 97)

Preheat the oven to 350°F (180°C).

Halve the tomatoes and put them in a baking dish. Add a little olive oil, salt, and pepper, and bake for 15 minutes.

Fill a large, deep pot with water and bring it to a boil. Cook the lobsters for 1 minute (see tip). Remove from the water and let cool. Cut the lobsters in half lengthwise and remove the stomach pouch at the top of the trunk and the intestinal tract in the tail, leaving the meat. Lay the lobsters, cut side up, in a separate baking dish.

Finely chop the basil and mince the garlic. Mix and add the lime juice and a generous splash of olive oil. Season with salt and pepper. Pour the sauce onto the lobster meat. Bake for 8 minutes or set them on the grill until the meat is opaque and firm to the touch. Do not turn the lobster over; this would waste the tasty juices. Pull legs and claws from the body with a twist and serve with lobster on a plate.

Cut the lettuce into large pieces and finely chop the chives. Put them in a large bowl. Add the warm tomatoes and the mayonnaise and mix well. The lettuce will wilt a little from the heat of the tomatoes (see tip). Serve the lobster and salad together.

TIP: Cooking lobster

First, place the live lobster in the freezer for 15 minutes. Cold has an anesthetic effect. Fill a large, deep pot with water and bring to a boil. When the water is at a full rolling boil, put the lobster in the water, head first. This way, it will be dead within seconds. If you think you hear it "squeal," I can reassure you that lobsters are totally incapable of squealing; the noise comes from air escaping from under the shell.

TIP: Salad with warm tomatoes

This salad is particularly surprising: With the heat of the tomatoes, the flavors mix much better and the lettuce wilts a little. Delicious and different.

Grilled Langoustines with Roasted Tomatoes

5 tomatoes

1 bunch basil

12 raw langoustines
(see tip)

3 sprigs flat-leaf
parsley

Preheat the oven to 200°F (100°C).

Bring a saucepan of water to a boil. Cut a small X in the bottom of each tomato, cutting through the skin but no deeper. Put the tomatoes in the boiling water for a few seconds, until the skin begins to curl around the incision. Remove from the water with a slotted spoon and run under cold water to cool. Peel the tomatoes: The skin should come off easily. Quarter the tomatoes and remove the seeds over a sieve set in a bowl to catch the liquid. Press on the seeds to extract more juice. Finely chop the basil and mix it with the tomato juice; add ¼ cup (60 ml) olive oil and season with salt and pepper. Arrange the tomatoes in a baking dish, round side up, and spoon the basil sauce over them. Bake for 30 minutes. Remove the tomatoes from the oven and increase the oven temperature to 350°F (180°C).

Cut the langoustines in half lengthwise; remove the intestinal tract and stomach pouch. Place them in a baking dish, cut side up.

Chop the parsley and mix it with 3 tablespoons olive oil and salt and pepper. Sprinkle this mixture over the langoustines. Bake for 5 to 10 minutes. The meat should be just barely opaque and tender.

Serve the langoustines and tomatoes straight from the baking dishes.

TIP: Langoustines
Langoustines are really haute cuisine. They are in the same family as lobster, but much better—more flavorful and tender. And just like lobsters, they are expensive. But when I see them fresh for sale (which is not often) I have to buy them. It is one of those little luxuries I cannot resist. You could replace them with shrimp or lobster, and the dish will be delicious as well, but if you try it with langoustines, you will not regret it.

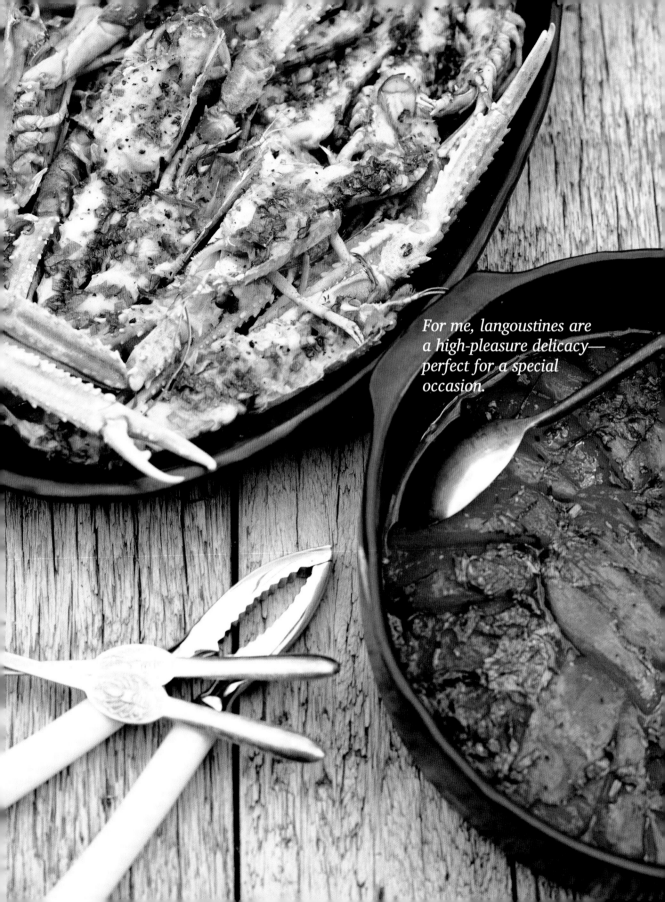

For me, langoustines are a high-pleasure delicacy— perfect for a special occasion.

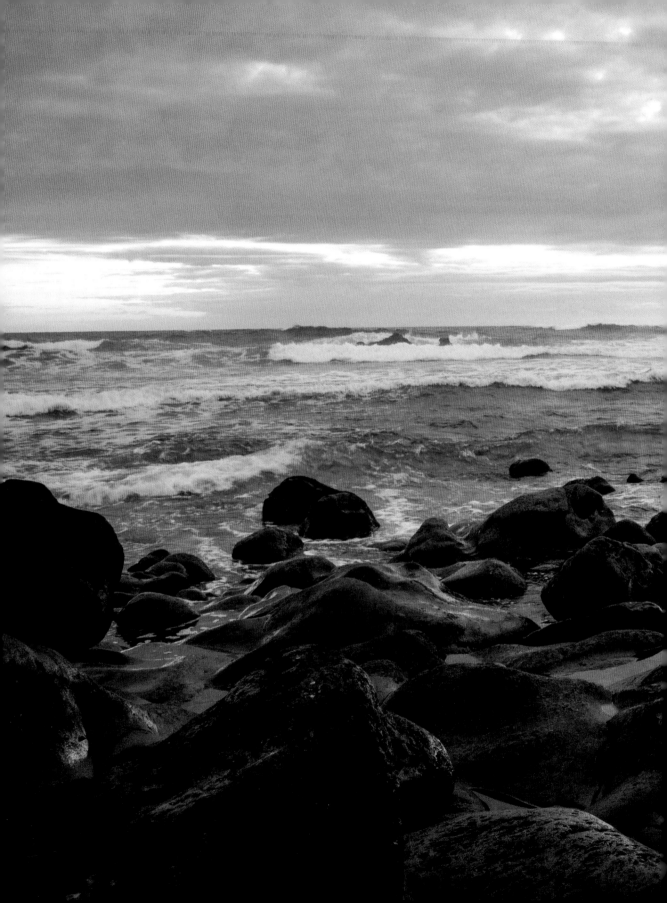

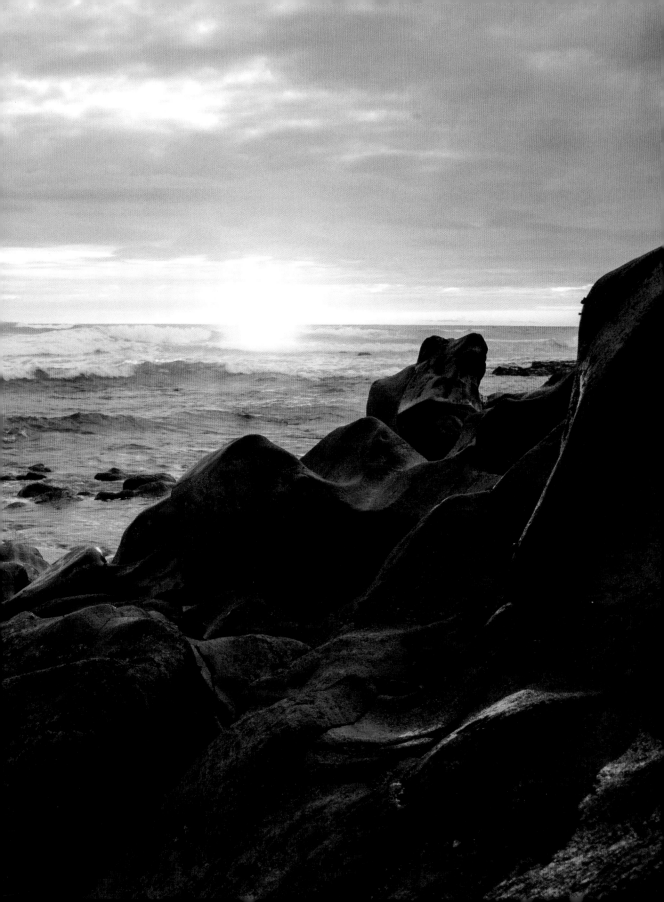

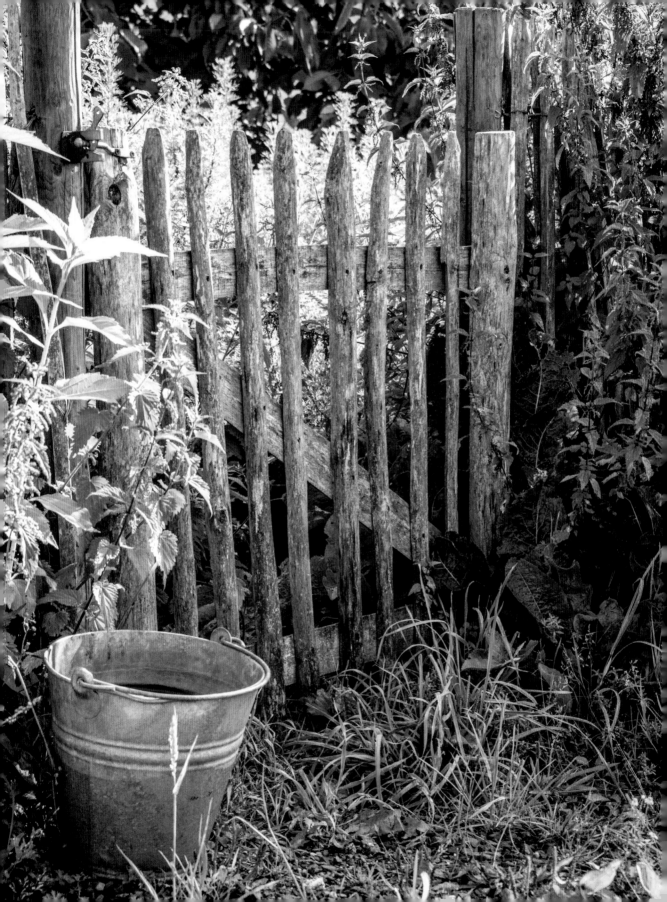

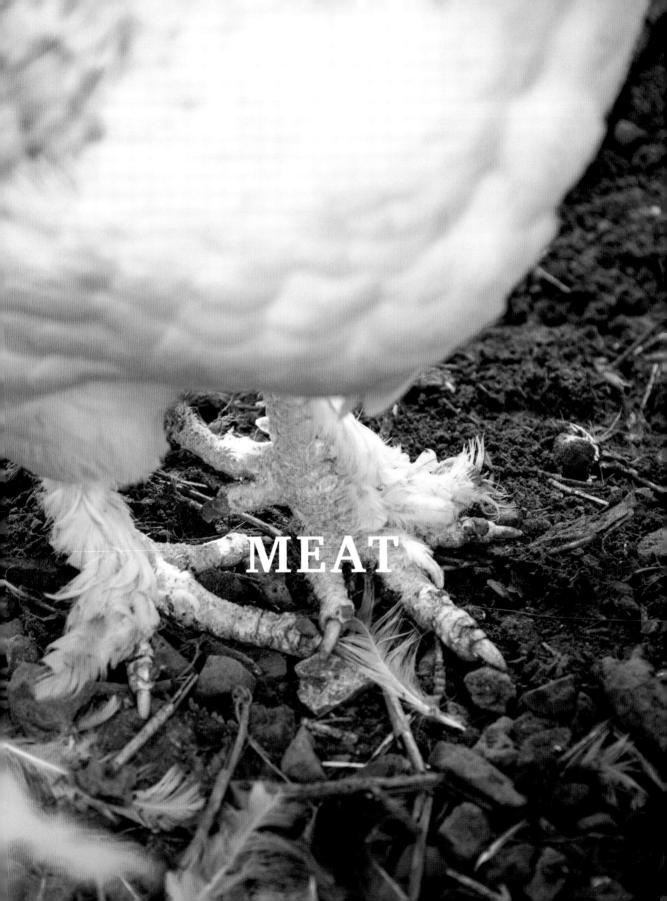

MEAT

Chicken Cabbage Rolls with Sesame-Soy Dipping Sauce

MAKES
10 to 12 rolls

PREPARATION
20 minutes

COOKING TIME
25 minutes

3 garlic cloves

1 (1-inch/2.5-cm) piece
fresh ginger

2 scallions

1 bunch cilantro

9 ounces (255 g) ground
chicken

6 outer leaves of 1 savoy
cabbage or green cabbage
(see tip)

For the sauce:

¼ cup (60 ml) toasted
sesame oil or olive oil

3 tablespoons soy sauce

juice of 1 lime

1 to 2 tablespoons toasted
sesame seeds (see page 135)

Chop the garlic, ginger, scallions, and cilantro. Knead them into the ground chicken just until combined (do not overmix).

Bring a saucepan of water to a boil. Put the outer leaves of the cabbage in the boiling water for 2 minutes (see tip). Blanch a maximum of three leaves at a time. Cut the cabbage leaves in half along the thick center rib, removing the rib. Place a small quantity of the chicken mixture in the middle of each leaf half, fold the sides in, and roll the leaf around the filling.

Bring about 1 inch (2.5 cm) of water to a simmer in a saucepan with a steamer insert or set a bamboo steamer on top. Place the rolls in the steamer, seam side down, and steam them for 15 to 20 minutes, until the filling is firm and cooked through.

Meanwhile, make the sauce: Mix the sesame oil, soy sauce, lime juice, and sesame seeds in a bowl.

Arrange the rolls on a serving dish and give everyone an individual bowl with some sauce. Serve with chopsticks.

TIP: Cabbage
Choose a large cabbage: The leaves will be larger and easier to handle. Making the rolls may be a little intimidating in the beginning, but have faith. Also, if the sides are not perfectly folded in, don't worry: The filling holds together well and will not fall out. If necessary, stick a toothpick in each roll to hold it together.

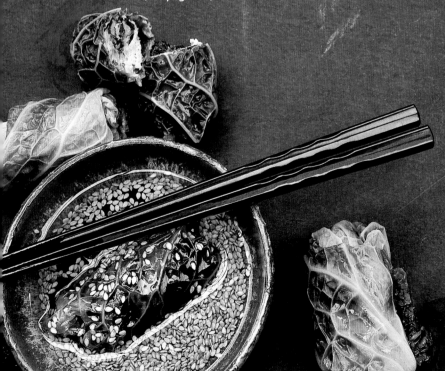

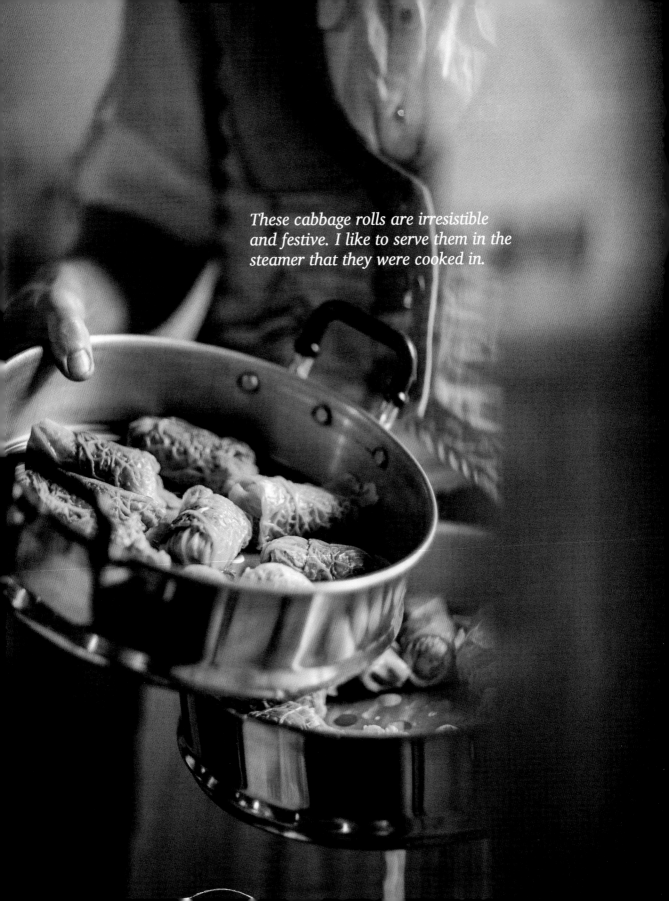

These cabbage rolls are irresistible and festive. I like to serve them in the steamer that they were cooked in.

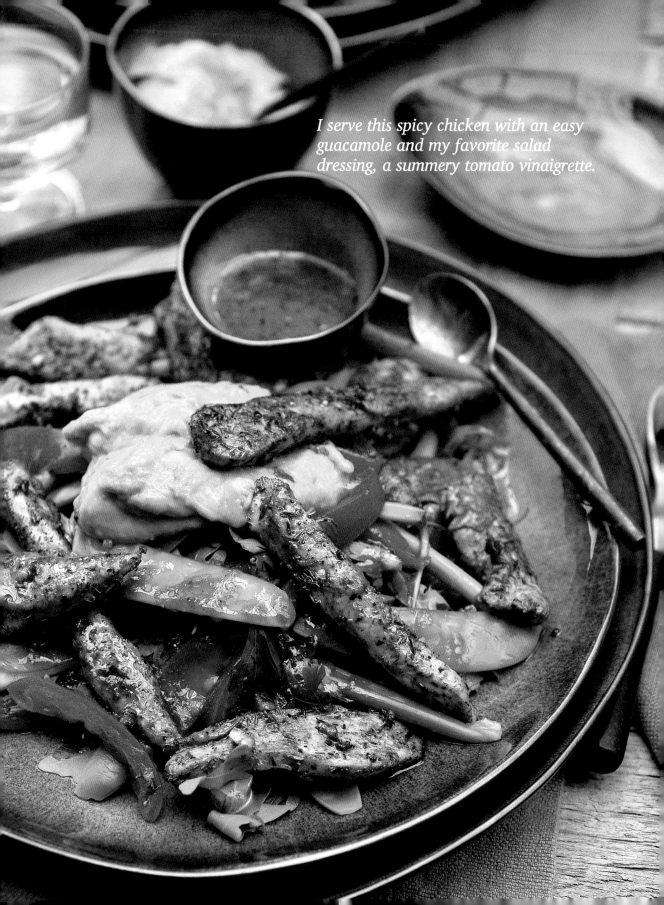

I serve this spicy chicken with an easy guacamole and my favorite salad dressing, a summery tomato vinaigrette.

Cajun Chicken Salad with Guacamole

2 (7- to 10½-ounce/
200- to 300-g)
boneless, skinless
chicken breasts

For the Cajun spice mix:

4 teaspoons sweet
paprika

3 tablespoons dried
thyme

2 garlic cloves, minced

pinch of cayenne
pepper

7 ounces (200 g) sugar
snap peas

4 tomatoes

1 ripe avocado

juice of 1 lime

arugula

Cut the chicken into long strips.

In a bowl, make the Cajun spice mix: Combine the paprika, thyme, garlic, cayenne, and some olive oil. Add the chicken and coat with the mixture. Let the chicken marinate for at least 5 minutes (see tip).

Bring a saucepan of water to a boil. Add a little oil and the peas and cook until al dente; drain well.

Quarter, core, and seed the tomatoes. Slice the tomatoes into thin wedges. Do this over a sieve and keep the juices for the vinaigrette (see tip, page 123).

Make a vinaigrette with the tomato juice, 2 to 3 tablespoons olive oil, and salt and pepper.

Halve, pit, and peel the avocado; put the flesh in a bowl and add the lime juice. Season with salt and pepper, and mash (see tip).

In a skillet over medium heat, cook the chicken in a bit of olive oil for 10 to 15 minutes, until cooked through.

Toss the tomatoes and peas with the arugula, and arrange them on plates. Divide the guacamole and chicken strips between the plates. Serve the vinaigrette separately.

TIP: Marinating

You can even start marinating the day before and leave it overnight in the fridge, which will make this more flavorful. But I am quite an impulsive cooker and even 5 minutes will do.

TIP: Guacamole

If you don't have time to make guacamole from scratch, you can use store-bought guacamole. In this recipe, I made a very simplified version; you are, of course, free to add chiles and fresh herbs if you wish.

SERVES
2

PREPARATION
20 minutes

COOKING TIME
20 minutes

Chicken and Zucchini Curry Soup

2 (7- to 10½-ounce/
200- to 300-g)
boneless, skinless
chicken breasts

1 bunch fresh Italian/
flat-leaf parsley or
cilantro (whichever
you prefer)

2 garlic cloves

2 white onions

¾ cup (180 ml)
coconut milk

3 tablespoons green
curry paste

1 large zucchini

Cut the chicken into small pieces. Finely chop the parsley.

Mince the garlic and finely chop the onions. Heat a little olive oil in a sauce-pan over medium heat. Add the garlic and onions and cook over low heat, stirring frequently. Do not let the onion turn brown; this would result in a brown soup.

Add the coconut milk, 2 cups (480 ml) water, the curry paste, and the parsley. Simmer for a few minutes. Mix well, then add the chicken and simmer until the chicken is cooked through.

While the soup is cooking, thinly slice the zucchini. Heat a little oil in a skillet over medium-high heat. Add the zucchini and cook until just tender, about 5 to 10 minutes. Season with salt and pepper.

Right before serving, add the zucchini to the soup. Enjoy!

I love the warm and inviting scent of curry that fills my house when I make this bright, fresh soup.

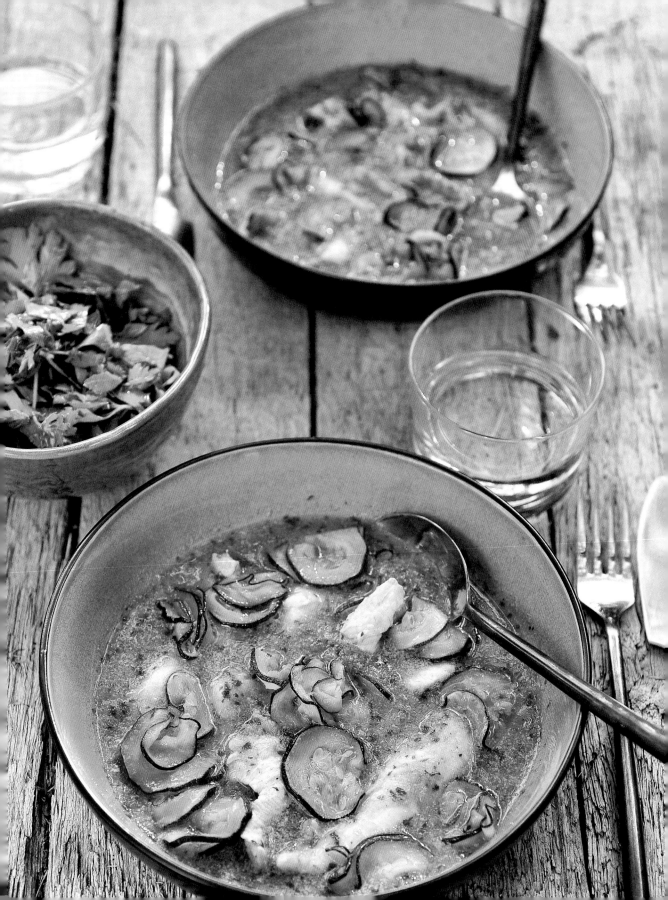

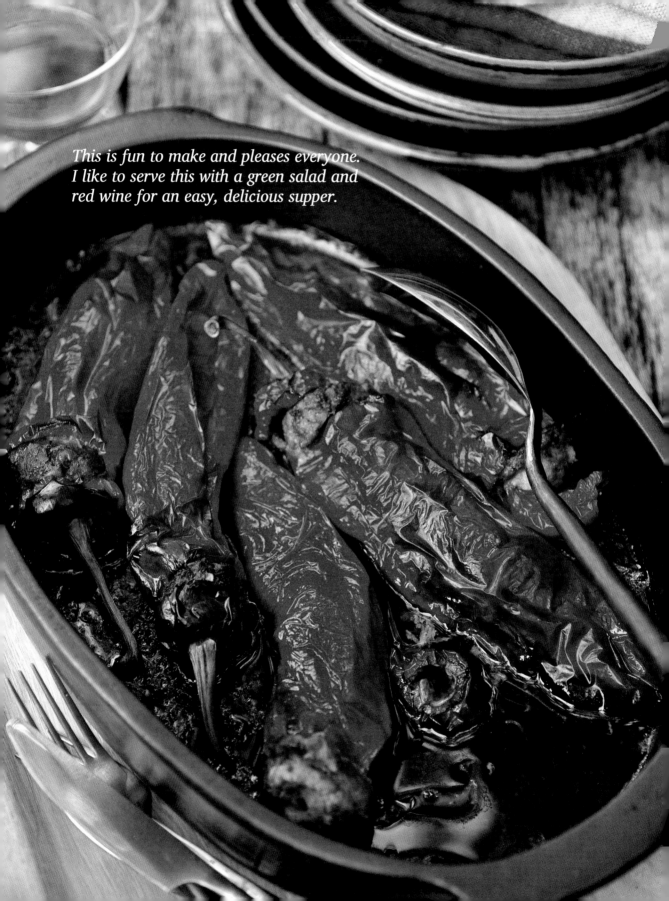

*This is fun to make and pleases everyone.
I like to serve this with a green salad and
red wine for an easy, delicious supper.*

Peppers Stuffed with Ground Chicken and Herbs

⅔ cup (150 g) green olives, pitted

10 sun-dried tomatoes in olive oil, drained

handful of fresh basil

handful of pine nuts

2 garlic cloves

1 pound (455 g) ground chicken (see tip)

4 large red bell peppers or poblano peppers

Preheat the oven to 350°F (180°C).

Finely chop the olives, sun-dried tomatoes, basil, pine nuts, and garlic. Add to a bowl with the ground chicken and a splash of olive oil. Season with salt and pepper and mix just until combined (do not overmix, see tip).

Cut just the tops off the peppers, reserving the tops, and carefully remove the seeds.

With the tip of a knife, cut a small notch at the bottom of each pepper, which will allow air to escape and should make filling narrow peppers easier. Using a small spoon, insert some stuffing into the pepper and push it down with the back of the spoon. Fill the peppers three-quarters full. (When you hold the pepper in front of a light you can see how full it is.)

Lay the peppers in a baking dish and arrange the caps around them. Bake for 30 minutes, until the peppers are tender and the chicken is cooked through, then serve.

TIP: Ground chicken

Ground chicken can be found in any supermarket. If you prefer to make it yourself, use the leg meat, because it is not as dry as breast meat and is more flavorful.

TIP: Don't use a food processor

If you use a food processor to make the stuffing, you lose all the texture in your meat and the mixture becomes too mushy. It is faster—that, I'll admit—but the end result suffers.

SERVES
2

PREPARATION
15 minutes

COOKING TIME
1 hour and 30 minutes

Thyme-Crusted Chicken with Fennel, Shallots, and Tomatoes

2 bunches thyme (see tip)

4 garlic cloves

juice of 3 lemons

1 large fennel bulb

2 chicken drumsticks

2 chicken leg quarters

8 shallots

8 tomatoes (see tip)

Preheat the oven to 350°F (180°C).

Strip the thyme leaves off the stems and put them in a food processor. Add the garlic, lemon juice, some salt, pepper, and a splash of olive oil and pulse to obtain a thick but fluid sauce.

Slice the fennel and arrange it in a single layer in a baking dish. Season with salt and pepper. Place the chicken on top. Pull off the papery outer layers of the shallots and place the whole shallots around the chicken; add the tomatoes. Coat the chicken with the thyme mixture; some of the sauce may cover the vegetables.

Cover the dish with aluminum foil and bake for 1 hour. Remove the foil and bake for another 30 minutes to obtain a nice golden brown color.

TIP: Thyme

Do not be frugal with the thyme, since it is the main flavor of this dish. Use at least two full bunches. The taste will not be overwhelming. The sauce must cover the chicken entirely.

TIP: Tomatoes

Yes, people often ask why I use tomatoes in so many of my recipes. The answer is: They are delicious, versatile, healthy, and beautiful. I would add them to all my preparations. However, if you are not a fan, you can simply leave them out. The fennel and shallots are the interesting ingredients in this dish.

This chicken dish is particularly flavorful, with tender fennel and shallots. This is a balanced, standout one-pan dinner.

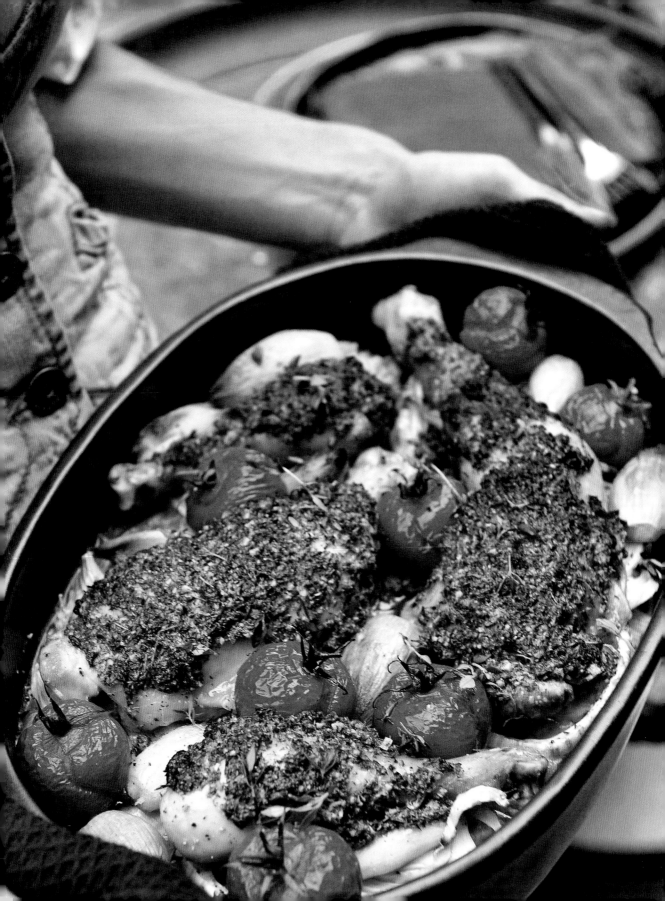

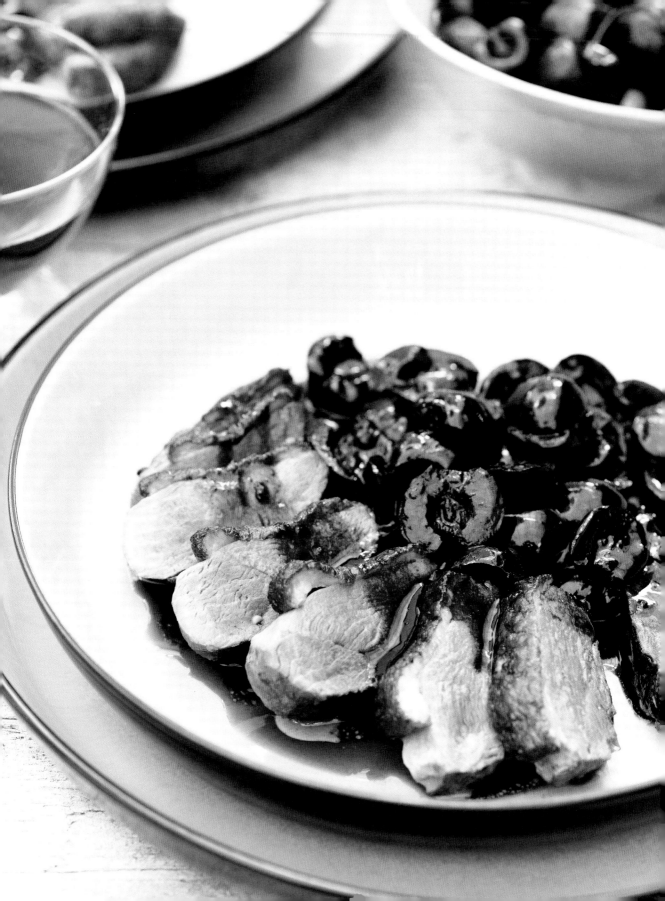

Duck Breast with Cherries

2 duck breasts

10½ ounces (300 g) sweet cherries

balsamic vinegar

Preheat the oven to 350°F (180°C).

Do not remove the fat from the breasts. Score the skin and fat on each breast at ¼-inch (6-mm) intervals without cutting through into the meat. In an ovenproof skillet over medium-high heat, cook the breasts fat side down for 4 minutes; the fat will soon begin to render. Turn the breasts over and cook for 3 to 4 minutes more. Season with salt and pepper and place the skillet in the oven for 7 minutes, or until the meat is cooked to a nice medium-rare.

Pit the cherries (see tip) and halve them. Heat a generous splash of olive oil in a skillet over medium heat. Add the cherries and cook until they release their juice, about 5 minutes. Add a splash of vinegar and let them stew for a few minutes. Season with pepper.

Cut the duck breasts into thick slices against the grain and set them on a serving platter. Arrange the cherries around them. Use the pan juices from the cherries as a sauce.

TIP: Pitting cherries
This is very easy to do with a cherry pitter—very handy if you have a lot of cherries. You will find cherry pitters in kitchen supply stores and online. If you don't have one, though, no problem—it will just take a little more elbow grease. Cut cherries in half and pull out the pits.

When I occasionally prepare fruit with meat, I always go for simple pairings, such as chicken with apples or this amazing combination of savory and sweet. It is so simple in every way that it is just perfect.

SERVES
4

PREPARATION
25 minutes

COOKING TIME
1 hour and 10 minutes

Roasted Rosemary Lamb, Tomatoes, and Carrots

1 bulb garlic

6 to 8 sprigs rosemary

1 (4-pound/2-kg) bone-in leg of lamb (see tip)

10 tomatoes

5 large carrots

leaves from a few sprigs fresh thyme

Preheat the oven to 350°F (180°C).

Peel all the garlic cloves and drop them into a food processor. Pull the rosemary leaves from the stems and add them to the food processor along with some salt, pepper, and a generous splash of olive oil. Pulse to obtain a thick, coarsely chopped mixture. Thoroughly coat the lamb with the garlic mixture. (If you don't have enough, make more!) Place the lamb in a baking dish.

Chop the tomatoes into large pieces, add salt, pepper, and olive oil, and arrange them around the meat. Cover the baking dish with a lid or aluminum foil. Bake for 40 minutes. Remove the lid or aluminum foil, return to the oven, and bake for 5 to 10 minutes more to allow the meat to brown (see tip). Remove the meat from the oven, cover, and let sit for 20 minutes. Leave the oven on.

While the lamb rests, thinly slice the carrots and put them in a baking dish. Give them a splash of olive oil and roast until soft, about 10 to 15 minutes. Stir frequently. Season with salt and pepper and fresh thyme.

Slice the meat and serve with the tomatoes and carrots.

TIP: Leg of lamb
I always ask my butcher to cut the bone loose and put it back in. Meats cooked with the bone have more flavor. After cooking, when I want to slice the meat, I first pull out the bone using a circular motion, which is quite easy to do.

TIP: How long in the oven?
If you like your meat medium-rare, count on about 10 minutes per pound (455 g) plus 20 minutes of resting time. This resting time is very important. It pulls the heat inward and redistributes the juices so that the meat will remain moist when sliced. Note that these times are only guidelines. Check frequently, until the lamb reaches your desired internal temperature (e.g., 130°F to 135°F or 55°C to 60°C for medium-rare).

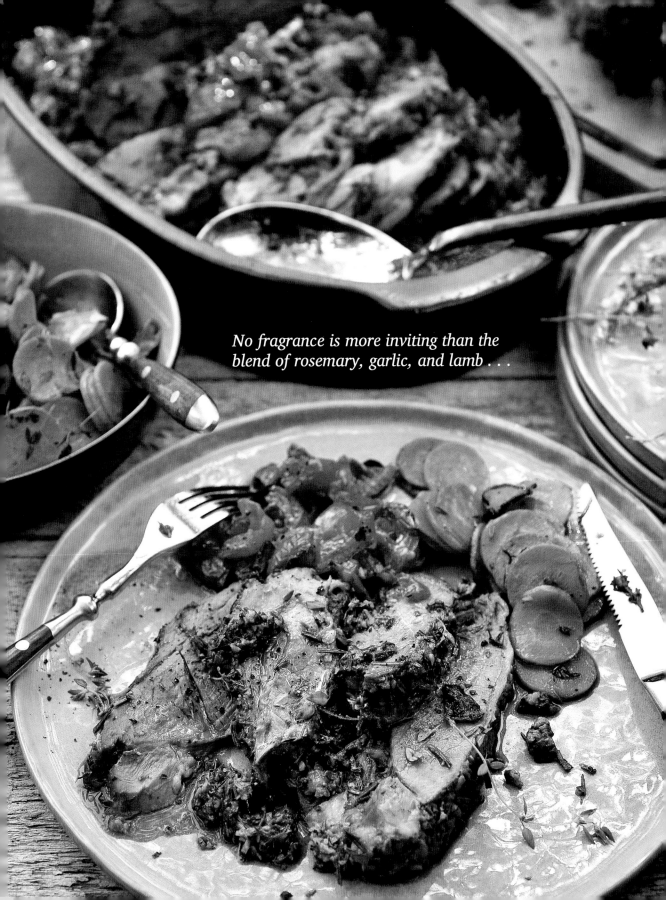

No fragrance is more inviting than the blend of rosemary, garlic, and lamb . . .

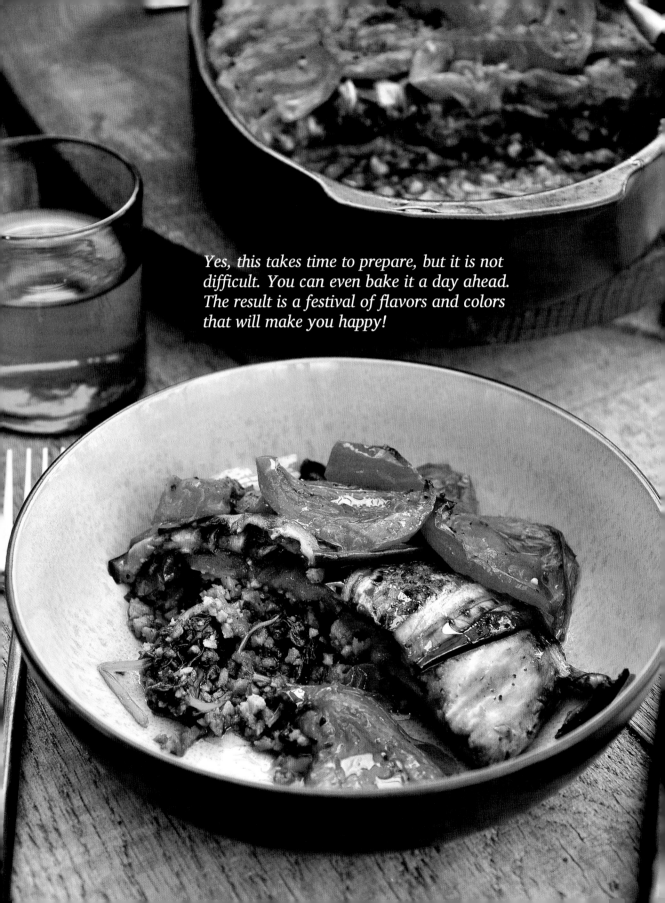

Yes, this takes time to prepare, but it is not difficult. You can even bake it a day ahead. The result is a festival of flavors and colors that will make you happy!

Ground Beef with Peppers and Eggplant

SERVES
2

PREPARATION
30 minutes

COOKING TIME
50 minutes

2 red bell peppers

6 tomatoes

2 globe eggplants

7 ounces (200 g) ground beef (or lamb or chicken)

7 ounces (200 g) spinach

Preheat the oven to 350°F (180°C).

Put the whole peppers in the middle of the oven on a baking sheet and roast for 25 to 30 minutes until blackened.

Quarter and seed the tomatoes (see tip). Place them skin side down in a baking dish; drizzle with olive oil and season with salt and pepper. Place the dish next to the peppers and bake for 30 minutes until skins are wrinkled and beginning to brown.

Slice the eggplant lengthwise into ⅜-inch- (1-cm-) thick slabs. Heat a grill pan over medium-high heat. Working in batches, add the eggplant and cook, turning frequently, until softened and browned. Transfer the eggplant to a plate, drizzle with olive oil, and season with salt and pepper. Repeat until all the slices are grilled.

Remove the bell peppers and tomatoes from the oven (keep the oven on). Toss the blackened bell peppers into a plastic bag and close it tight. Set aside until cool enough to handle.

Meanwhile, heat a little olive oil in a skillet over medium-high heat. Add the meat and cook, stirring to break up the clumps, until browned. Add the spinach and cook until the spinach wilts and the meat is cooked through. Season with salt and pepper.

Remove the bell peppers from the bag and peel them. Cut them in half, discard the seeds, and slice the peppers.

Spoon the spinach and meat mixture into a casserole dish. Next, add the roasted pepper slices. Then add a layer of eggplant slices and finish with the tomatoes, skin side down. Cover the dish with aluminum foil and bake for 20 minutes until bubbling.

TIP: Tomato juice
For baking, I prefer to seed the tomatoes, but I don't discard the pulpy centers. I pass them through a sieve and push the juices out. Then I either drink the tomato juice or make a delicious vinaigrette by simply adding a little olive oil and salt and pepper.

Ground Beef and Tomato Bake with Cauliflower Topping

½ head cauliflower

3 yellow onions

3 carrots

9 ounces (255 g) cherry tomatoes

3 garlic cloves

14 ounces (400 g) ground beef

Preheat the oven to 350°F (180°C).

Cut the cauliflower into florets. Dice the onions and carrots. Halve the tomatoes.

Bring a saucepan of water to a boil. Add the cauliflower, garlic, a generous splash of olive oil, and salt and pepper. Cook until the cauliflower is tender.

Heat a little olive oil in a skillet over medium-high heat. Add the onions and carrots and cook until tender. Add the ground beef and cook, stirring frequently and breaking up the meat, until it is browned. Season with a little salt and pepper. Add the tomatoes. Cook for about 3 minutes, then transfer to a baking dish.

When the cauliflower is tender, drain in a colander and return the pot to medium heat. Add a nice splash of olive oil and briefly sauté the cauliflower florets. Mash the cauliflower, preferably with a potato masher so as to keep a little texture. Add olive oil and mix. The more olive oil you add to the mash, the smoother it will be (see tip). Spoon the cauliflower over the vegetable mixture.

Bake for 15 to 20 minutes until cauliflower topping is browned, then serve.

TIP: Reheating
You can prepare this dish a day in advance and keep it in the refrigerator. Reheat it in the oven for 30 minutes before serving.

TIP: Don't be afraid of olive oil
Looking at the total number of calories or the total fat content is simply not the right way to determine if food is healthy or unhealthy. Think of nuts, vegetable fats rich in polyphenols, whole yogurt, and avocados . . . all foods that are good for our health. So don't skimp on the olive oil—it is flavorful, satisfying, and good for you.

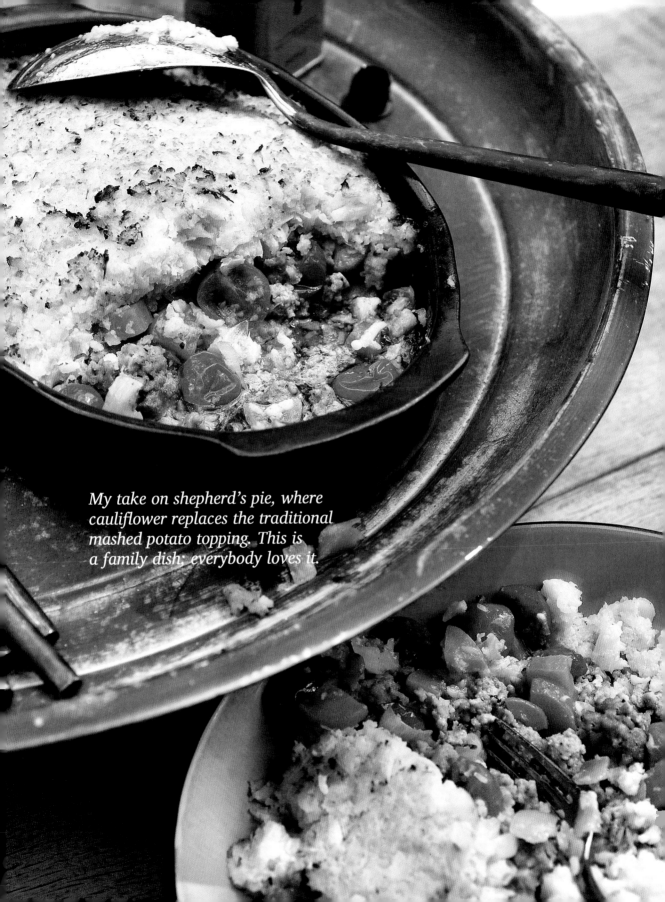

My take on shepherd's pie, where cauliflower replaces the traditional mashed potato topping. This is a family dish; everybody loves it.

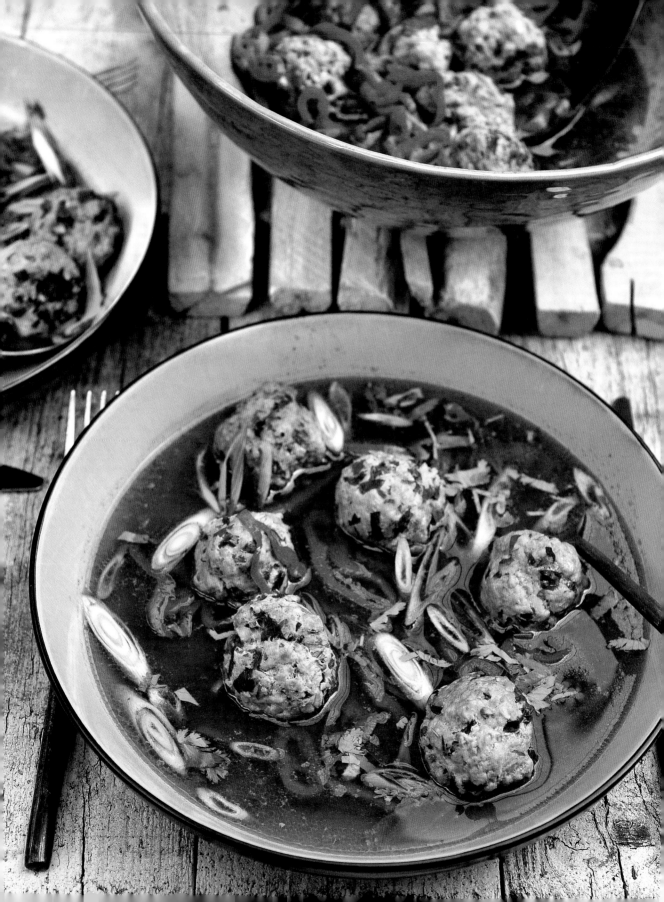

Meatballs in Ginger-Soy Broth

3 garlic cloves

1 (1½-inch/4-cm) piece fresh ginger

1 bunch cilantro

10½ to 14 ounces (300 to 400 g) ground beef

2 red bell peppers

½ cup (120 ml) soy sauce

2 scallions

Mince the garlic and ginger and finely chop the cilantro. Add them to a bowl with the meat and season with a little salt and black pepper. Mix just until combined (do not overmix). Roll the mixture into balls about 1 to 1½ inches (3 to 4 cm) in diameter. (They will shrink during cooking.)

Cut the peppers into thin rings. Heat a splash of olive oil in a skillet over medium-high heat and cook the bell peppers until tender. Add 2½ cups (600 ml) water and the soy sauce. Season with pepper. Before adding salt, taste the mixture, since soy sauce is already salty.

Bring the broth to a boil and add the meatballs. Simmer until they are cooked through (see tip).

Meanwhile, thinly slice the scallions on an angle. Sprinkle them over the soup right before serving.

TIP: Are the meatballs done?

I would suggest cooking them for 7 to 15 minutes. If you really want to be sure, take one out and cut it open.

These delicious, tender meatballs are ideal for sharing with a group; simply double or triple the recipe.

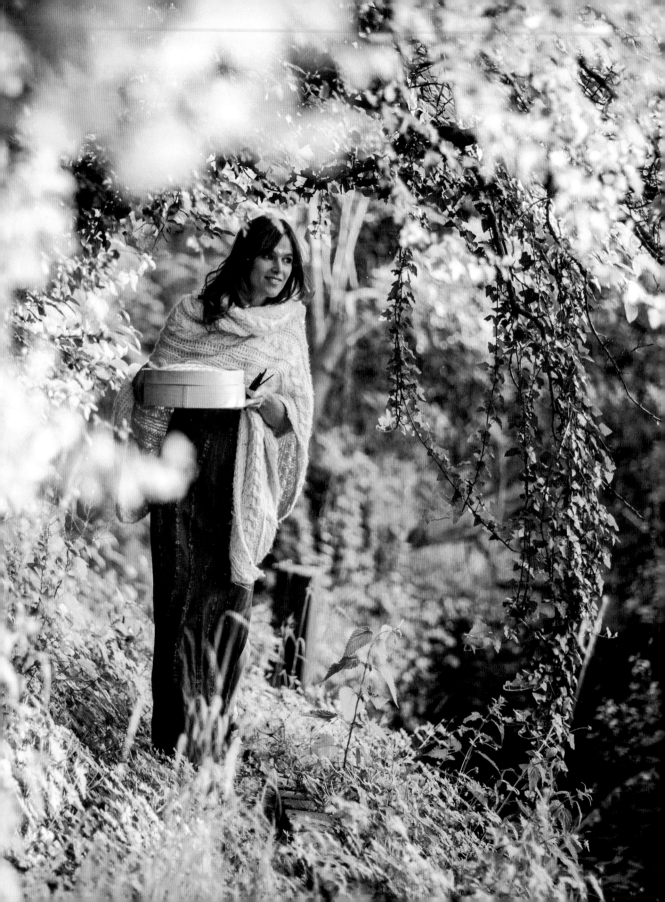

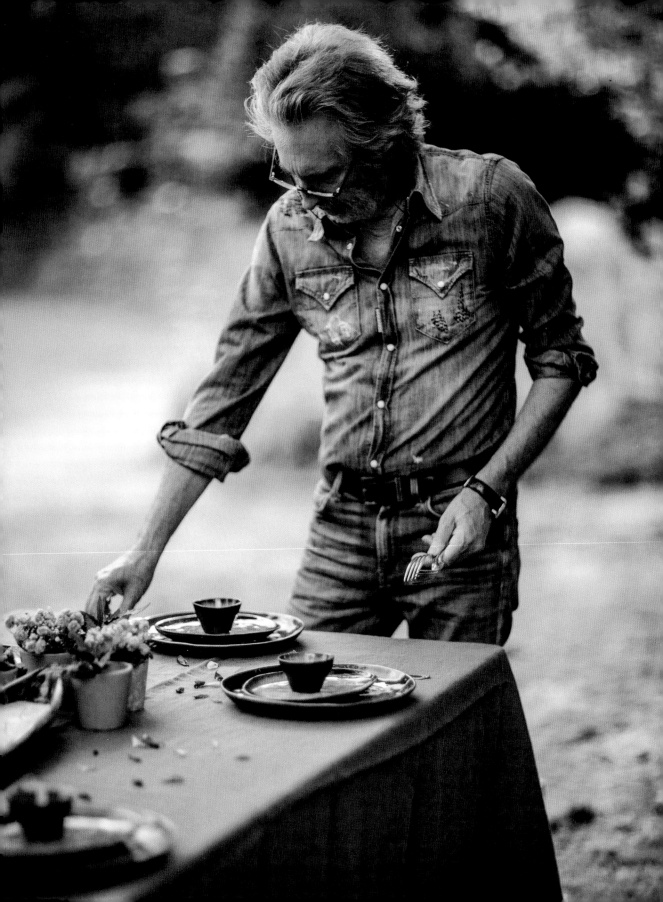

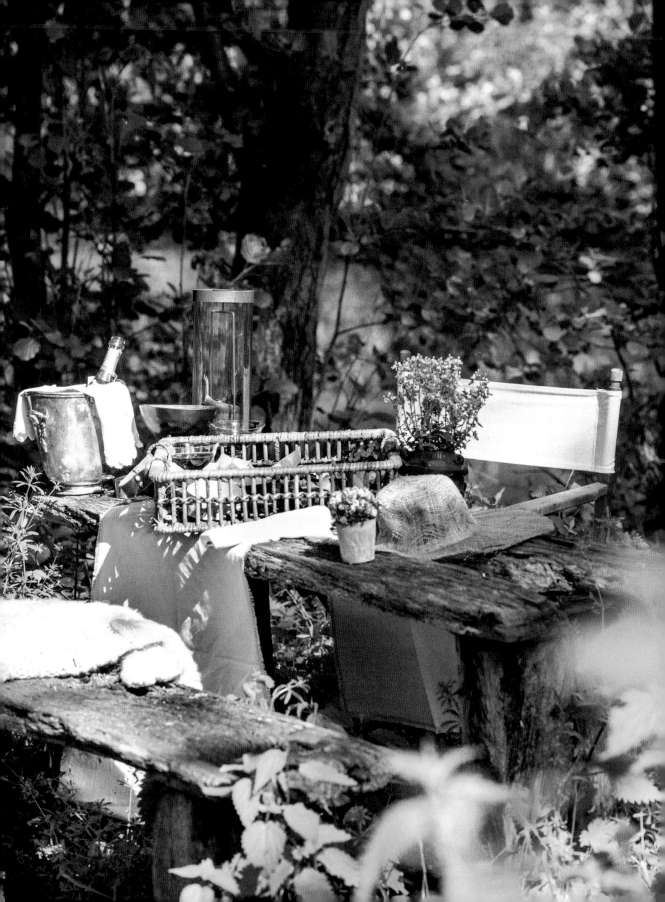

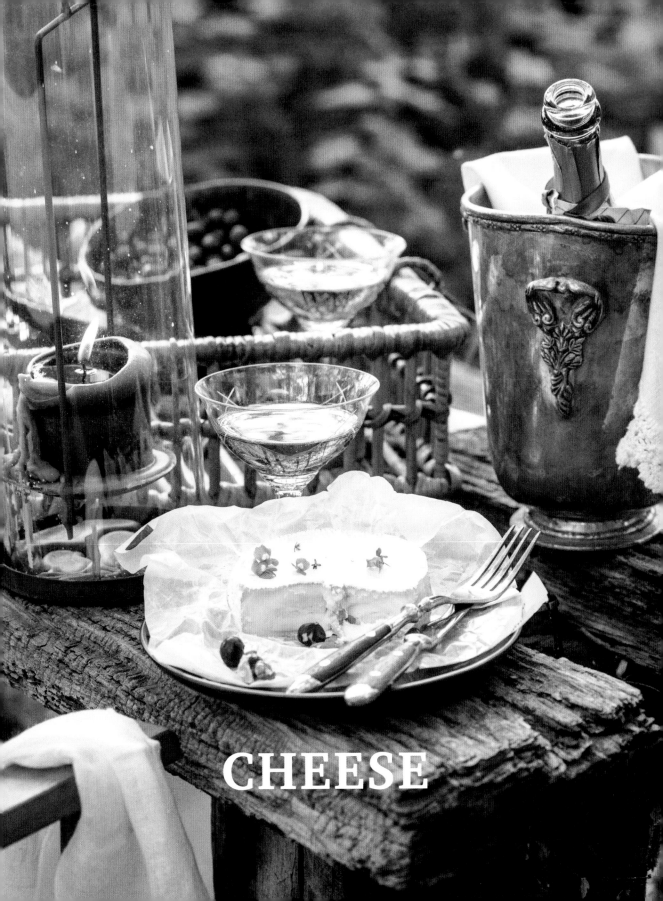

CHEESE

MAKES
about 20 chips

PREPARATION
3 minutes

COOKING TIME
10 to 15 minutes

Parmesan Chips

⅔ cup (65 g) grated Parmesan cheese

½ cup (65 g) mixed seeds (see tip)

Preheat the oven to 350°F (180°C). Line a baking sheet with parchment paper.

In a bowl, mix the cheese and seeds. Spoon small mounds of the mixture onto the prepared baking sheet, leaving some space between them. Do not flatten the mounds. Bake for 10 to 15 minutes. Check often: the chips should be light brown, but certainly not dark brown.

Remove from the oven and let cool before removing the chips from the paper and serving.

TIP: Mixed seeds

If you have prepared my fruit breakfast (see page 182), you already have a jar of mixed seeds in stock. Flax, chia, and pumpkin seeds: A mix of these three seeds is already plenty. However, you can certainly try sesame, hemp, and others.

One of the most popular snack recipes I make, these chips are so easy to prepare and so delicious.

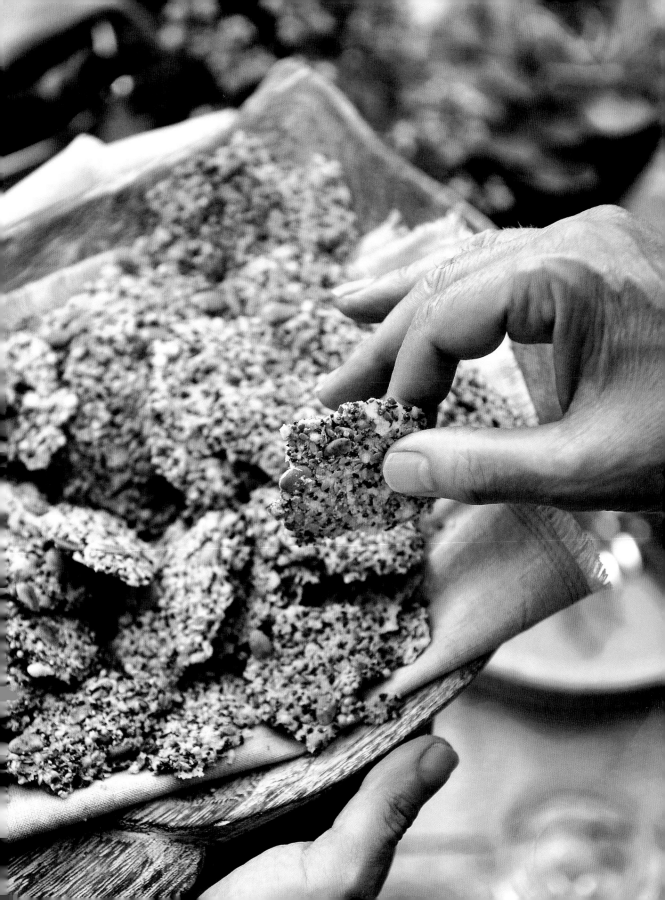

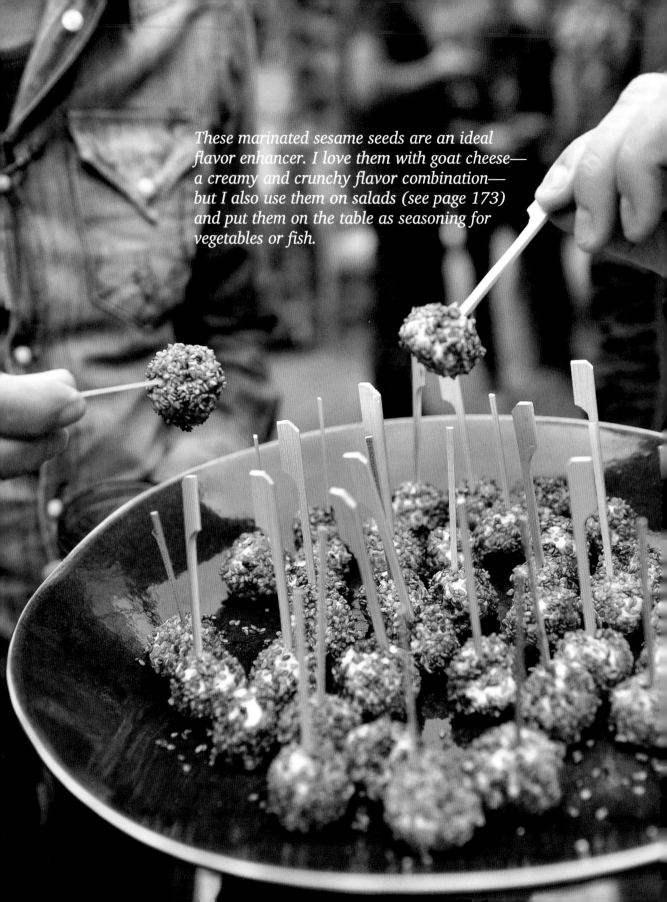

These marinated sesame seeds are an ideal flavor enhancer. I love them with goat cheese—a creamy and crunchy flavor combination—but I also use them on salads (see page 173) and put them on the table as seasoning for vegetables or fish.

MAKES
15 to 20 balls

PREPARATION
10 minutes

MARINATING
at least 15 minutes

COOKING TIME
6 to 10 minutes

Goat Cheese Bites with Marinated Sesame Seeds

2 to 3 ounces (60 to 80 g) sesame seeds (natural or toasted, see tip)

5 tablespoons (75 ml) soy sauce

7 ounces (200 g) soft goat cheese

Put the sesame seeds in a small bowl and pour over just enough soy sauce to cover them. Marinate for at least 15 minutes and up to 24 hours (see tip).

Preheat the oven to 350°F (180°C). Line a baking dish with parchment paper.

Drain the marinated sesame seeds and then spread them on the prepared baking dish. Bake for 6 to 10 minutes (see tip).

Make small balls of cheese and roll them in the sesame seeds. Serve them with toothpicks.

TIP: Toasted or natural sesame seeds
I love to use toasted sesame seeds in this recipe instead of natural sesame seeds, because they already have more of the toasted flavor.

TIP: Marinated sesame seeds
If you can marinate the seeds for the full 24 hours, they become more flavorful (but don't leave them any longer than a day). I usually marinate sesame seeds the evening before I need them.

TIP: Toasting sesame seeds
Check the seeds frequently to make sure they're not burning. Let them dry evenly and become crispy. They should not become dark brown; take them out when they are lightly browned. If necessary, reduce the oven temperature and let them roast a little bit more. Make extras as you can keep them for a few days on a piece of waxed paper in a cool place and use them in other dishes. If they lose their crunch, put them back in the oven for a few minutes.

Gazpacho with Basil-Cheese Crisps

5 tomatoes

¼ fennel bulb

1 generous bunch basil

1 teaspoon sweet paprika

2 tablespoons sherry vinegar

¾ cup (70 g) grated Parmesan cheese

Preheat the oven to 350°F (180°C). Line a baking sheet with parchment paper or aluminum foil.

Core and chop the tomatoes. Chop the fennel. Put the tomatoes and fennel in a food processor, add a few basil leaves (reserve the rest for the cheese crisps), the paprika, and vinegar, and season with pepper. Pulse until the vegetables are finely chopped. Add water until you reach a souplike consistency. Process until smooth.

Finely chop the remaining basil and mix with the cheese and a generous amount of black pepper.

Arrange the cheese-basil mixture in small, long mounds about ⅜ inch (1 cm) thick on the prepared baking sheet. No need to flatten them.

Bake for 5 to 7 minutes, or until they turn light brown. Remove from the oven and let cool.

Right before serving, sprinkle a few drops of olive oil into the soup. Serve the crisps with the tomato soup.

In the summer, I like to serve this soup with small ice cubes. It is a refreshing, memorable snack or a light prelude to a larger meal.

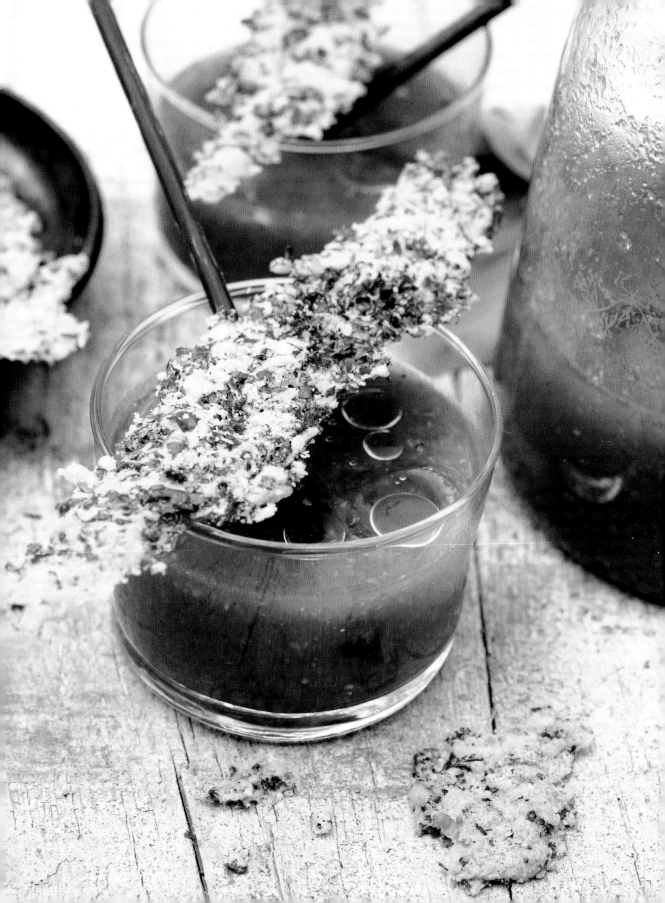

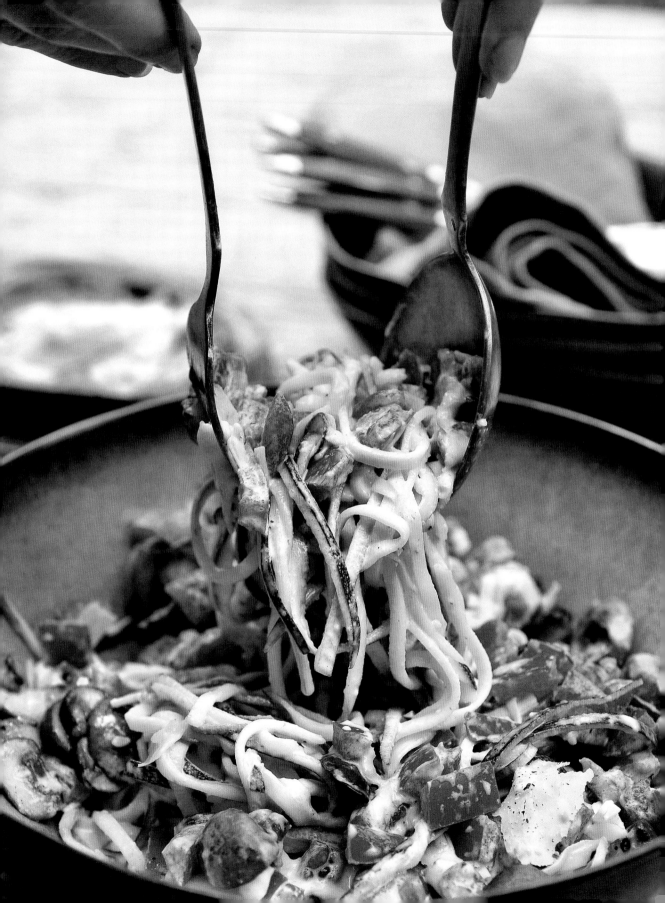

Zucchini Noodles with Tomatoes, Mushrooms, and Parmesan Sauce

2 or 3 zucchini

4 tomatoes

8 ounces (225 g) button mushrooms

For the sauce:

1 cup (240 ml) heavy cream

½ cup (50 g) grated Parmesan cheese, plus a handful of shaved Parmesan

Using a julienne peeler, slice the zucchini lengthwise into ribbons. Put the ribbons in a bowl and sprinkle with olive oil. Set aside to marinate and soften.

Seed and finely chop the tomatoes.

Chop the mushrooms. Heat a little olive oil in a skillet over medium-high heat. Add the mushrooms and cook until they are lightly browned. Season with salt and pepper.

Stir together the cream and grated cheese in a saucepan. Bring just to a simmer over medium heat and cook a few minutes until you obtain a thick sauce. Season with salt and pepper.

Reserve some tomatoes and mushrooms for garnish. Gently fold the vegetables into the cheese sauce, and garnish with the reserved tomatoes and mushrooms. Finish with the Parmesan shavings.

This healthy combination of vegetables is as rich and flavorful as a creamy pasta.

SERVES
2

PREPARATION
10 minutes

COOKING TIME
15 minutes

Halloumi and Spinach Curry

about 3 tablespoons
green curry paste
(see tip)

7 ounces (200 g)
halloumi cheese

1 tablespoon cumin
seeds

14 ounces (400 g)
spinach

In a medium bowl, stir together the curry paste and 2 tablespoons olive oil. Cut the halloumi cheese into cubes and fold them into the curry paste mixture. Heat a skillet over medium heat and add the halloumi mixture. Cook for 5 to 7 minutes, until the cubes just start to melt.

In a separate dry skillet, toast the cumin seeds until they just begin to smoke and release their aroma (see tip). Add a splash of olive oil and the spinach. Stir until the spinach is totally cooked. Season with pepper and a little salt (the cheese is already very salty).

Spread the spinach on plates and top with the curried cheese cubes.

TIP: Green curry

There are many different types of green curry paste, from mild to very hot. If you like heat, buy your curry paste from an Asian food store; the standard grocery store variety will be milder. It is always preferable to taste beforehand, and adjust the quantity accordingly.

TIP: Cumin seeds

This typical Indian practice of heating the cumin seeds in a dry pan results in a very fragrant spice. You could also use cumin powder; the flavor is not as strong. In that case, add the cumin after cooking the spinach.

Inspired by the traditional Indian curry
saag paneer, this take features tender
spinach, set off by salty halloumi.

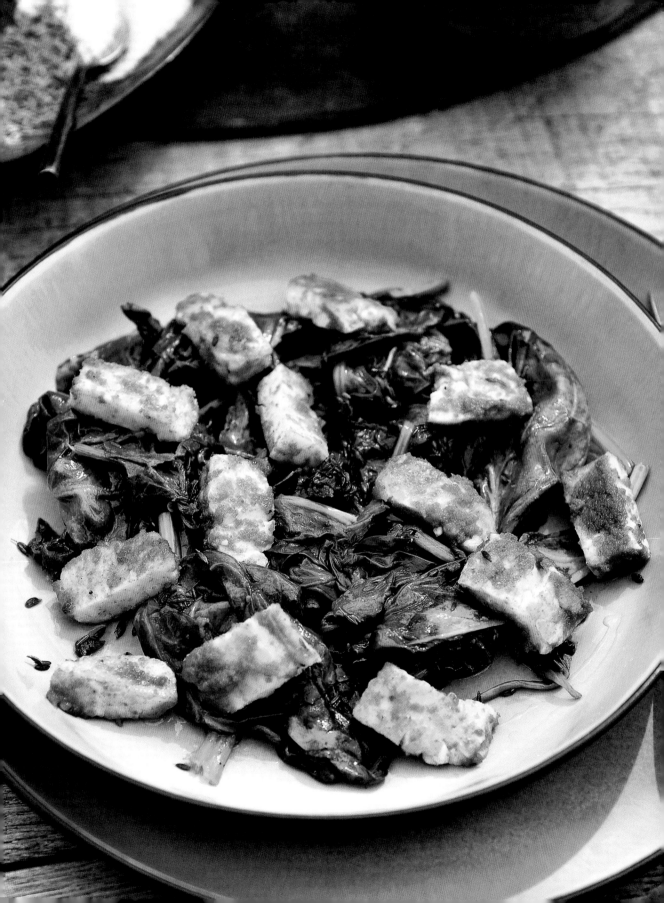

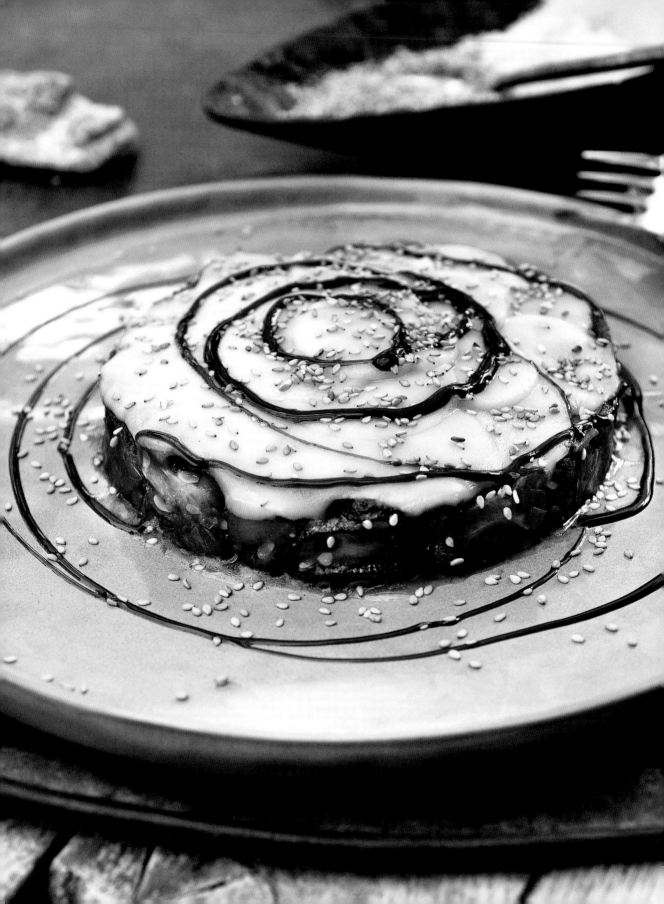

SERVES
2

PREPARATION
10 minutes

COOKING TIME
10 minutes

Zucchini, Tomato, and Cheese Carpaccio

2 tomatoes

1 zucchini

2 tablespoons capers, drained

5 thin slices of cheese (choose your favorite cheese that melts, such as Gouda)

toasted sesame seeds (see page 135)

balsamic syrup (see tip)

Core and chop the tomatoes. Cut the zucchini into thin slices. Heat a splash of olive oil in a skillet over medium-high heat. Add the zucchini. After a few minutes or when the zucchini is soft, add the tomatoes. Season with pepper and a little salt. Cook for 2 or 3 minutes more, until the tomato is softened but not saucy, then add the capers and simmer for a few minutes.

Place the cheese slices on top of one another and use a small ring mold or biscuit cutter to cut rounds of cheese.

Place a large ring mold on each plate and fill it first with the vegetable mixture. Place a cut round of cheese over the vegetables. Finish with the sesame seeds and balsamic syrup.

TIP: Make it at home
If you cannot find balsamic syrup, you can make it yourself with normal balsamic vinegar. Boil the vinegar in a saucepan and let it reduce until you get a thick syrup.

The presentation of this dish is elegant and memorable—a true match for its rich flavors. The cheese slowly melts over the warm veggies. Irresistible!

SERVES
2 to 4

PREPARATION
20 minutes

COOKING TIME
40 minutes

Eggplant and Zucchini "Lasagna"

2 zucchini

2 eggplants

6 tomatoes

½ red bell pepper

14 ounces (400 g) spinach

1⅔ cups (405 ml) ricotta

1 (6.3-oz/180-g) jar basil pesto

handful of shredded cheese

Preheat the oven to 350°F (180°C).

Slice the zucchini, eggplants, and tomatoes. Line a baking sheet or grill pan with aluminum foil. Brush the foil with olive oil and sprinkle with salt and pepper. Arrange the vegetable slices on the prepared pan. Brush the tops of the vegetables with olive oil and season with salt and pepper. Bake for 30 minutes (see tip) until they are soft and tender, and the zucchini and eggplant are light brown (keep the oven on).

Meanwhile, dice the bell pepper. Heat a splash of olive oil in a skillet over medium heat. Add the pepper and sauté until soft, then add the spinach. When the spinach is wilted, add the ricotta and season with pepper and a little salt. Cook for a few minutes more, then remove from the heat.

Arrange the zucchini slices in a baking dish (see tip). Brush with 2 or 3 tablespoons of the pesto. Then, spoon a layer of the ricotta-vegetable mixture over the top. Next add the eggplant slices. Brush with 2 or 3 tablespoons of the pesto, and follow with another layer of the ricotta-vegetable mixture. Finish with a layer of tomatoes. Garnish with the shredded cheese—Cheddar, Emmantaler, Gruyère, or Gouda are a few suggestions.

Bake the lasagna for 20 minutes, allowing the juices and flavors to mix and until the top starts to brown, then serve.

TIP: Vegetables in the oven
If the vegetable slices take up too much space, you may need to use up to three baking dishes or bake them in several batches. In any case, you don't have to keep the vegetables warm, because they will all go back into the oven before serving.

TIP: Layers
It actually doesn't matter how many layers you build, but always begin with zucchini and always end with tomatoes. The order of the intermediate layers is not important.

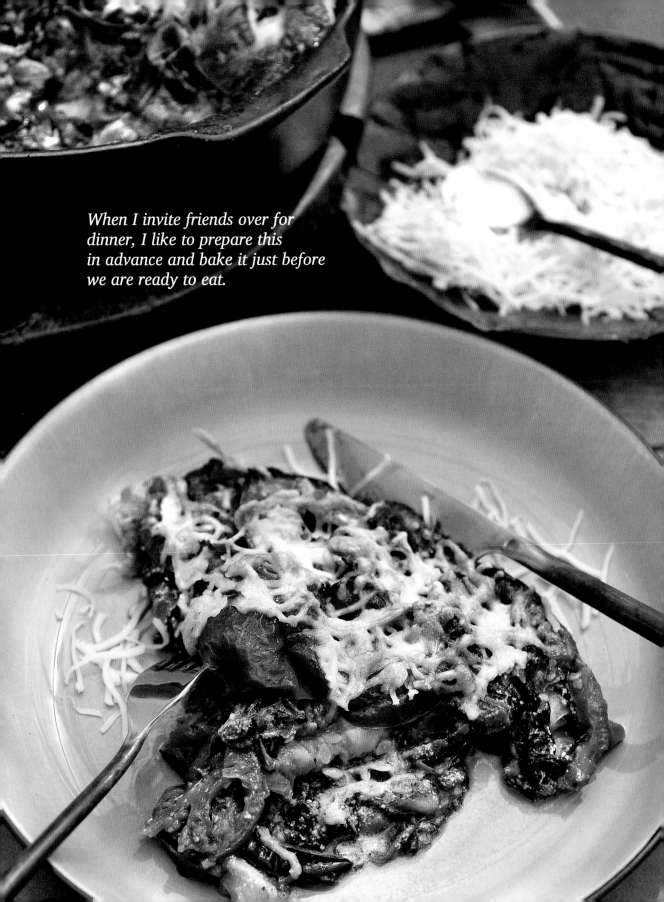

When I invite friends over for dinner, I like to prepare this in advance and bake it just before we are ready to eat.

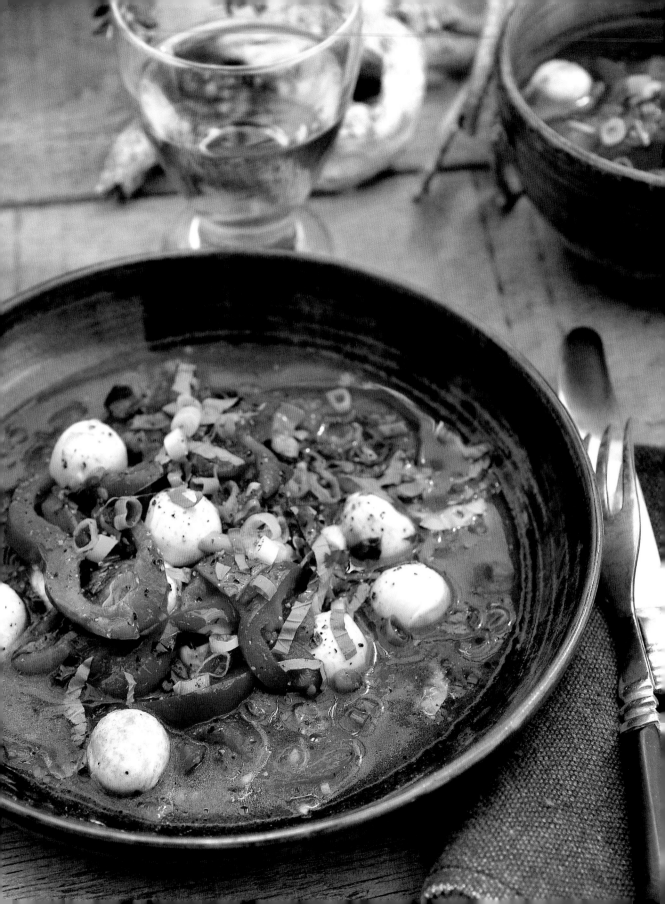

SERVES
2

PREPARATION
10 minutes

COOKING TIME
15 minutes

Tomato and Bell Pepper Soup with Mozzarella

2 red bell peppers

2 garlic cloves

4 large tomatoes

1 bunch basil

4 scallions

7 ounces (200 g) small balls of fresh mozzarella

Cut the bell peppers into thin rings; mince the garlic. Heat a splash of olive oil in a skillet over medium heat. Add the bell pepper and garlic and cook for 5 minutes.

Meanwhile, core the tomatoes and cut them into thick slices. Add them to the skillet and cook for 10 minutes, until the tomatoes are soft. Add about 1 cup (240 ml) water and season with a little salt and pepper. Bring to a simmer and cook for a few minutes more.

Finely chop the basil and scallions.

Remove the pan from the heat and add the basil, scallions, and cheese. Divide between two soup bowls and serve.

These fresh Mediterranean flavors are perfect for a quick, summertime lunch.

Warm Feta with Tomatoes and Olives

1 (7-ounce/200-g) block feta cheese

handful of mixed olives (see tip)

4 tomatoes

Preheat the oven to 350°F (180°C).

Halve the feta and place each piece in an individual ramekin or small oven-proof dish (see tip).

Divide the olives between the dishes. Cut a few tomato slices; core and quarter the rest. Lay the tomato slices over the feta and arrange the quartered tomatoes around it. Season all with a generous amount of pepper and season the tomatoes with a little salt (the feta and olives are already salty). Sprinkle olive oil over the whole dish, including the tomatoes. Bake for 30 minutes until the feta is tender and soft and starts to brown, then serve.

TIP: Serving
You can prepare this in one single dish; however, serving in individual ramekins is more practical and also much more attractive.

TIP: Which olives?
All olives are suitable for this: marinated or not, pitted or not. There is only one rule: If you like them cold, you will also like them hot. Actually, cooked olives are tastier!

The feta melts in your mouth—a delicious and straightforward dish. I like to pair this with a simple green salad for a satisfying weeknight meal.

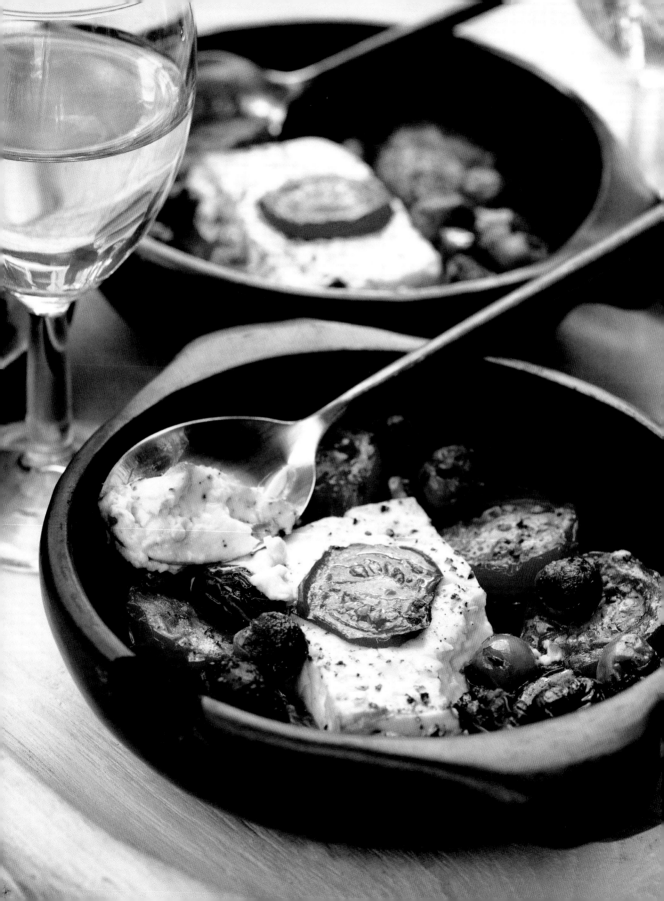

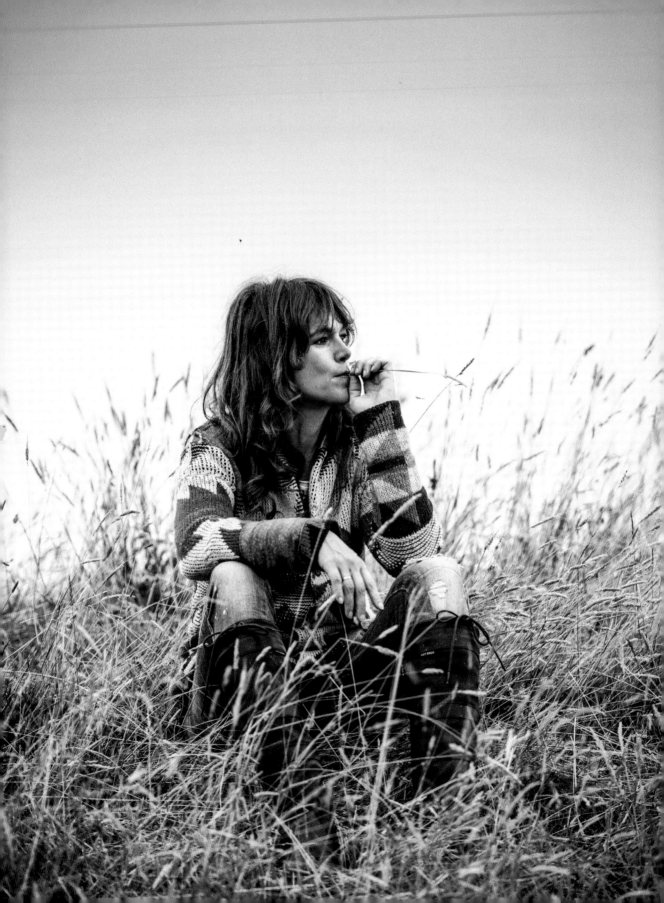

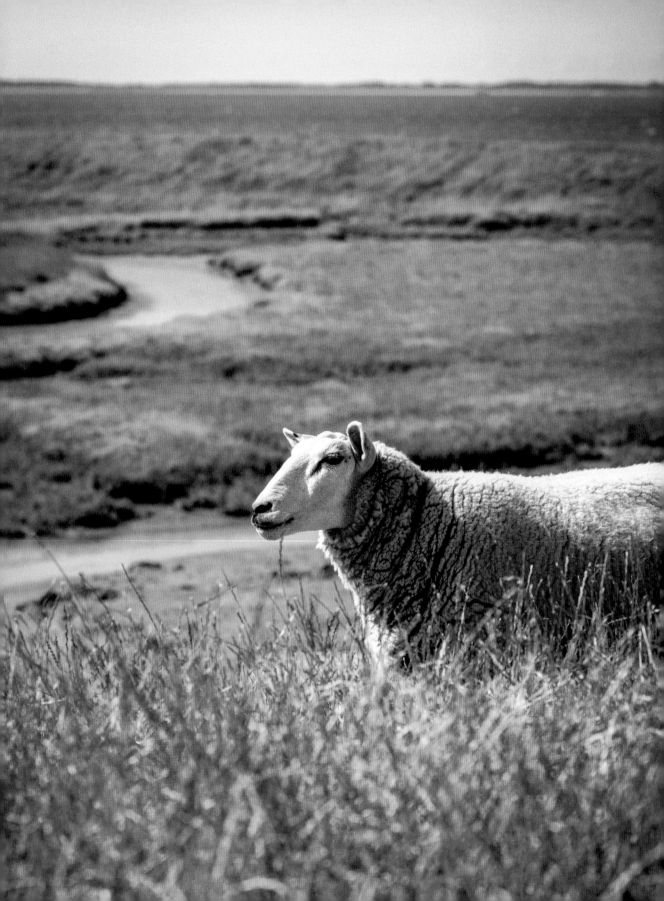

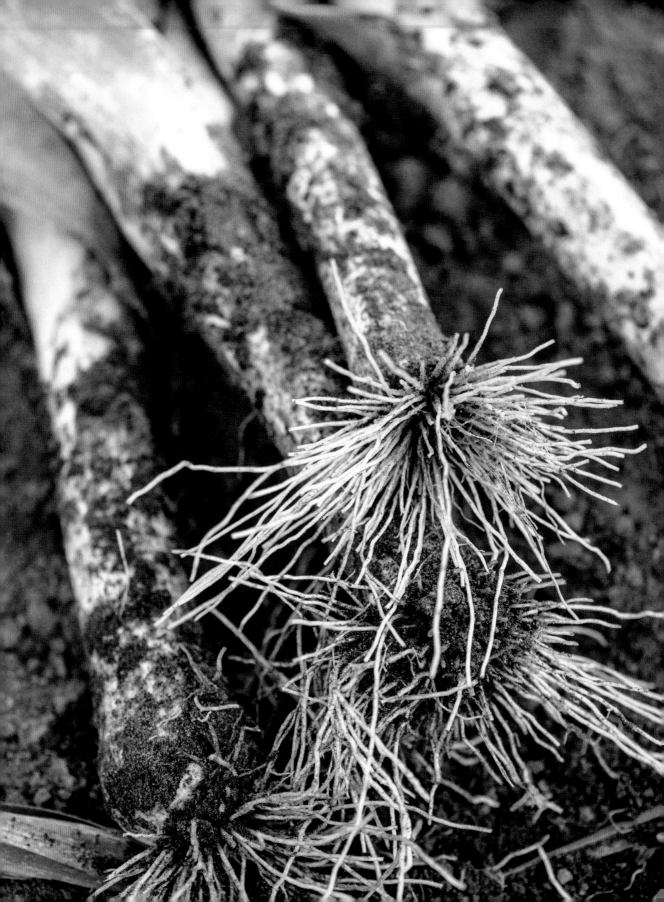

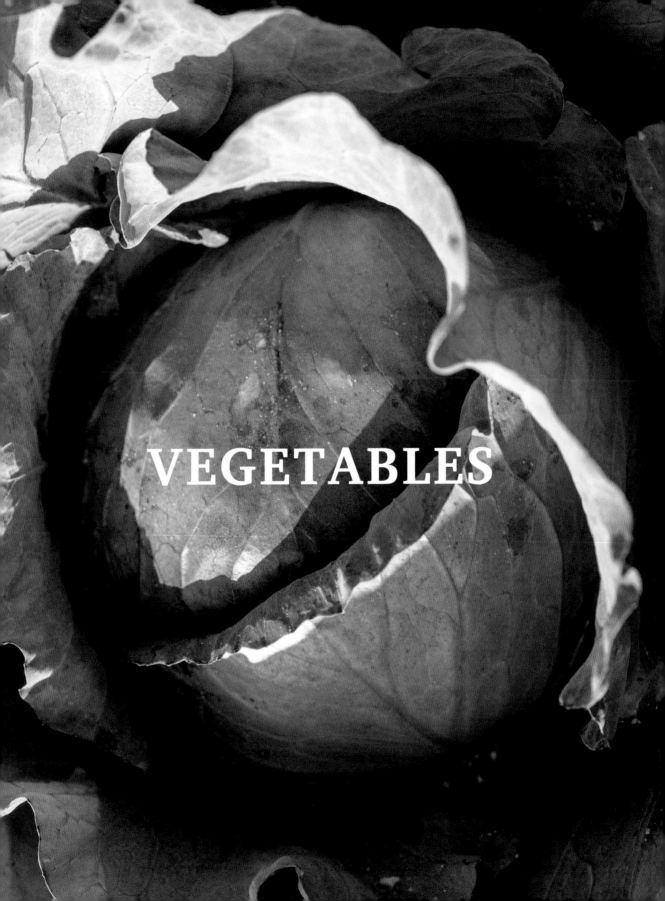

VEGETABLES

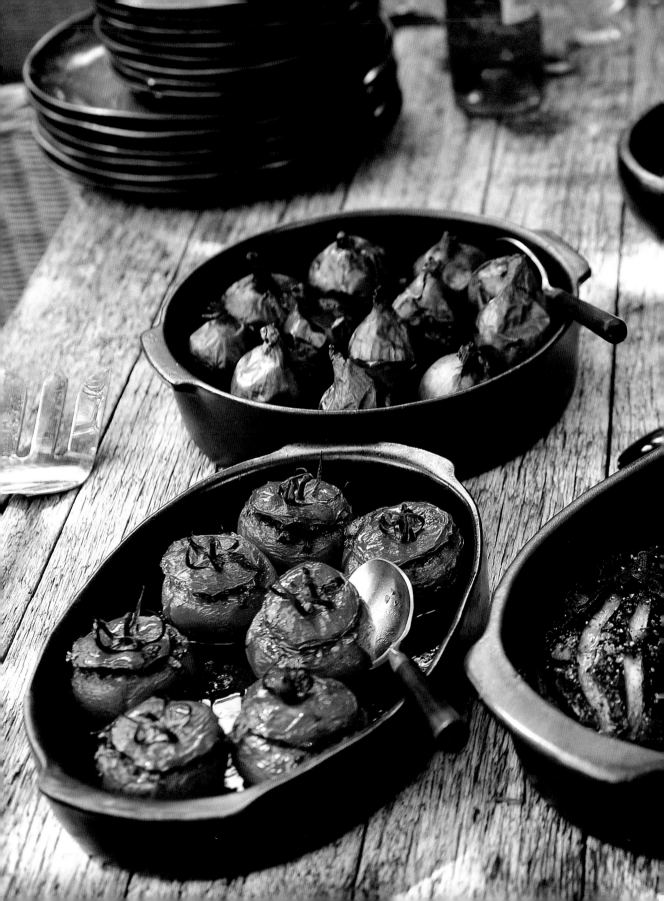

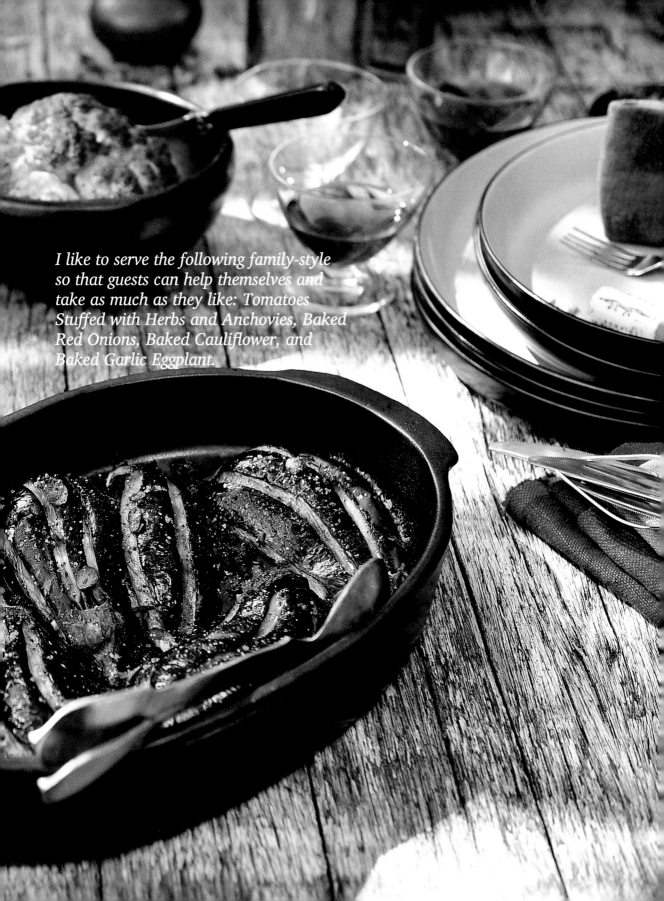

I like to serve the following family-style so that guests can help themselves and take as much as they like: Tomatoes Stuffed with Herbs and Anchovies, Baked Red Onions, Baked Cauliflower, and Baked Garlic Eggplant.

Baked Red Onions

PREPARATION
1 minute

COOKING TIME
40 to 60 minutes

4 red onions

You'll be surprised how one single ingredient can make such a memorable side.

Preheat the oven to 350°F (180°C).

Place the onions in a baking dish so they stand upright against one another. You don't need to remove the outer papery layers. Don't add any oil. Regardless of the onion sizes, bake for 40 to 60 minutes. The onions should be butter-soft inside. You can trim the onion a little bit after cooking for a nice presentation

TIP: Grilling

This onion dish is also very easy to prepare on the grill. The outer layers will blacken, but inside, the onions will have a beautiful red color and a buttery texture that is truly surprising.

Tomatoes Stuffed with Herbs and Anchovies

PREPARATION
10 minutes

COOKING TIME
15 to 20 minutes

8 anchovy fillets

handful of fresh basil

1 generous bunch flat-leaf parsley

4 tomatoes on the vine

These tomatoes pair well with fish.

Preheat the oven to 350°F (180°C).

Finely chop the anchovy fillets and herbs; add ¼ cup (60 ml) olive oil and season with pepper (the anchovies are already salty). Slice off the tops of the tomatoes (reserve the tops) and hollow out the tomatoes with a small spoon. Fill them with the herb-anchovy mixture and replace the tops.

Arrange the tomatoes in a baking dish and bake for 15 to 20 minutes until the tops are browned, then serve.

TIP: Sauce

When you plate the dish, use the cooking juices as a sauce.

Baked Cauliflower

PREPARATION
5 minutes

COOKING TIME
30 minutes

1 head of cauliflower

1 heaping tablespoon ras el hanout

People love this simple recipe. It is marvelous with any of the meat dishes in this book.

Preheat the oven to 350°F (180°C).

Place the whole cauliflower in a large pot and add water to cover. Lightly season with salt, pepper, and a generous splash of olive oil. Bring to a boil and cook for 10 minutes.

Meanwhile, in a medium bowl, combine the ras el hanout with ½ cup (120 ml) olive oil and a generous amount of pepper.

Drain the cauliflower. Put it in a baking dish and brush the seasoned oil all over. Bake for 20 minutes, brushing the cauliflower with more seasoned oil after 10 minutes, until golden brown on the outside and tender on the inside.

Serve the cauliflower whole at the table.

Baked Garlic Eggplant with Sun-Dried Tomatoes

PREPARATION
15 minutes

COOKING TIME
30 minutes

2 globe eggplants

4 garlic cloves

6 sun-dried tomatoes in olive oil

I just love eggplants. After I discovered how easy and delicious they are to prepare, I can't stop cooking them!

Preheat the oven to 350°F (180°C).

Peel lengthwise strips of skin from the eggplant (see tip). Cut the eggplant in half lengthwise. Leave the crown on. Put the eggplant halves in a single layer, cut side down, in a baking dish.

Thinly slice the garlic and mince the tomatoes. In a small bowl, make a sauce with 5 tablespoons olive oil, some pepper, and a little salt. Add the garlic and tomatoes. Coat the eggplants with the sauce and let them soak in the olive oil. Bake for 30 minutes until the skins wrinkle and they are tender on the inside, then serve.

TIP: Tracing lines in the eggplant

Use a small knife or a vegetable peeler with a small blade. Start from the stem end and trace to the bottom. The lines not only make the dish more beautiful, but also allow the eggplant flesh to absorb the flavorful olive oil more easily. If you want to add a colorful—and healthy—accent, you can add a teaspoon of turmeric to the sauce. The contrast between the eggplant's black skin and the yellow lines is striking.

MAKES
20 rolls

PREPARATION
15 minutes

COOKING TIME
7 to 10 minutes

Brick Pastry Rolls with Olive and Sun-Dried Tomatoes Tapenade

10 sheets brick pastry (see tip)

handful of toasted sesame seeds (see page 135)

½ cup (150 g) black olive tapenade (see tip)

½ cup (150 g) olive and sun-dried tomato tapenade

Preheat the oven to 350°F (180°C).

Take a round brick sheet and cut it in half. Brush one side with olive oil and sprinkle with sesame seeds. Spread 3 tablespoons of the black olive tapenade along the cut edge of the brick sheet. Tightly roll up the sheet, starting with the tapenade edge. Place the roll on a baking sheet lined with parchment paper. Fill and roll the rest the same way, filling half the rolls with olive tapenade and half with sun-dried tomato tapenade. If you prefer smaller rolls, cut the sheet in half again and adjust the quantity of tapenade.

Bake for 7 to 10 minutes, or until the rolls turn light brown and crispy.

TIP: Brick sheets

Brick dough (also brik or warqa) originates from the Middle East—it is a very thin sheet made of wheat flour. People who are allergic to gluten should avoid these. Work with the dough one sheet at a time, and leave the rest in the package or under a humid towel—the dough dries very quickly since it is so thin. If you can't find it, you could use thin spring roll wrappers instead. But choose a good brand, one that is not heavily processed, with the fewest unnatural ingredients. The longer the rolls are, the more impressive they are to serve. The rolls pictured are about 10 inches (25 cm) long.

TIP: Tapenade

If I don't have much time to cook, I have no problem using store-bought olive tapenade. Although I have to say that making it yourself is really not that much work. Buy your favorite olives and sun-dried tomatoes marinated in oil. In a food processor, mix the olives with a little olive oil, garlic, and fresh herbs. Divide the tapenade between two bowls and add the sun-dried tomatoes to one bowl so you have two different flavors.

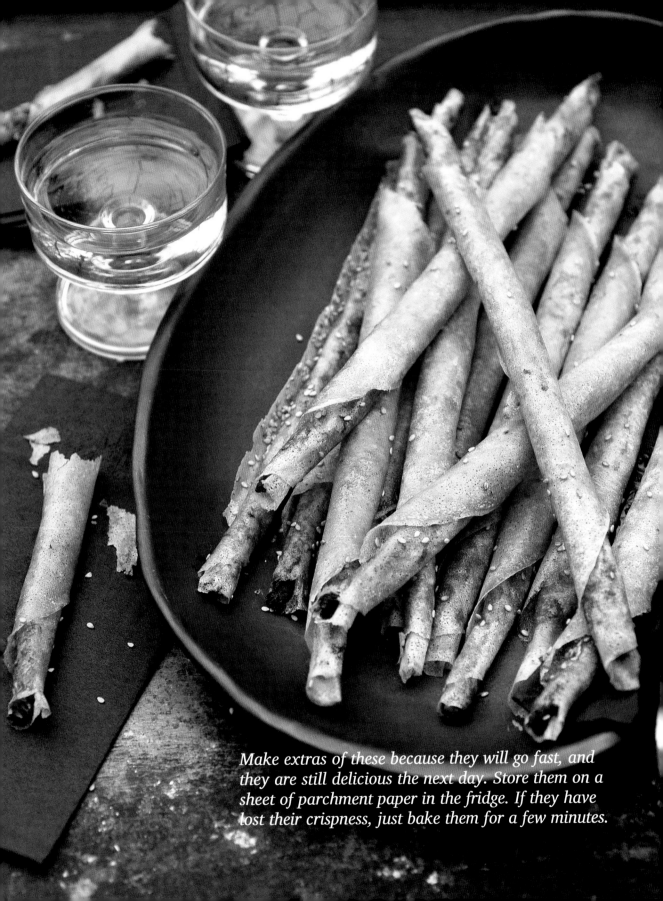

Make extras of these because they will go fast, and they are still delicious the next day. Store them on a sheet of parchment paper in the fridge. If they have lost their crispness, just bake them for a few minutes.

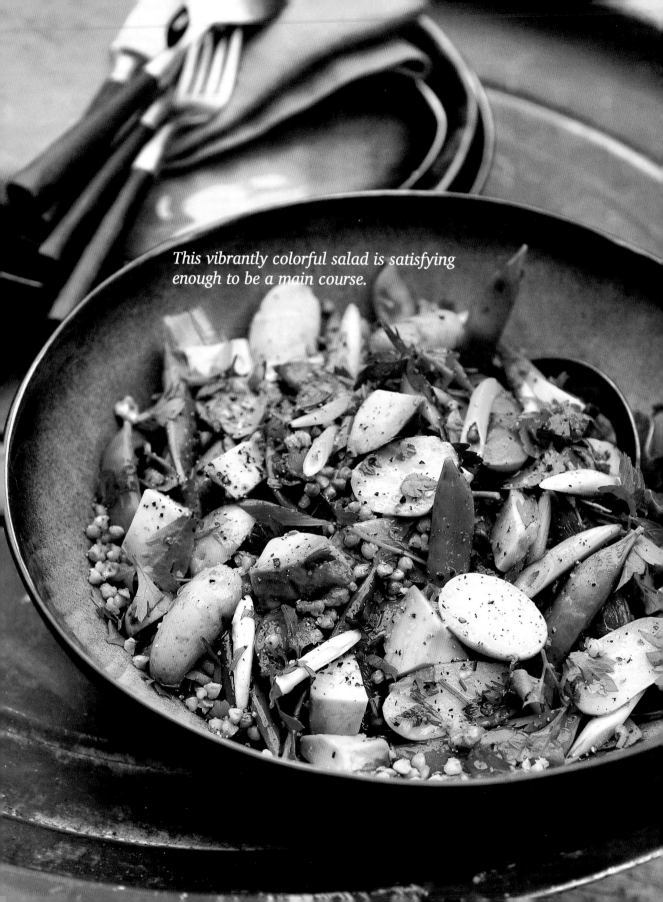

*This vibrantly colorful salad is satisfying
enough to be a main course.*

Buckwheat and Potato Salad

⅔ cup (110 g) whole buckwheat groats (see tip)

10 baby potatoes (see tip)

7 ounces (200 g) sugar snap peas

1 avocado

4 scallions

arugula or fresh herbs

Rinse the buckwheat. Put it in a saucepan with twice its volume of water and bring to a boil. Reduce the heat to a simmer and cook for about 15 minutes, or until tender.

Meanwhile, put the potatoes in a saucepan with enough water to cover and bring to a boil. Cook until fork-tender, about 12 minutes. Remove the potatoes from the water with a slotted spoon and add the peas. Cook for just a few minutes, until al dente, then drain.

Halve the potatoes and let them cool. Peel, pit, and chop the avocado and chop the scallions.

In a serving bowl, mix the peas, avocado, scallions, arugula, potatoes, and buckwheat. Season with salt and pepper. For me, the best way to dress this salad is with nothing but a little olive oil.

TIP: Buckwheat

Although buckwheat looks like a grain, it is not; it's something called a pseudo-grain. Buckwheat, amaranth, quinoa—all are pseudo-grains that have recently come into the spotlight. Like quinoa, buckwheat contains essential amino acids and is typically less refined than other grains. Buckwheat is gluten-free; it doesn't elevate blood sugar as much a conventional grains; it is a source of fiber, magnesium, potassium, phosphorus; and vitamins B_1 and B_6. Although buckwheat and quinoa contain a lot of other nutrients, they remain con-centrated carbohydrates (more than 10 percent of their content), so I prefer not to combine them with concentrated proteins (meat and fish), only with vegetables.

TIP: Potatoes

Eating potatoes every once in a while is fine, especially if you combine them with vegetables. This way, you eat fiber and the carbohydrates are not absorbed as quickly. If you let potatoes cool, the process results in the creation of an insoluble carbohydrate that is not digested by our enzymes but is a probiotic, meaning food for bacteria in the large intestine. This helps cultivate healthy intestinal flora.

SERVES
2 to 4 as an appetizer
or side dish

PREPARATION
10 minutes

COOKING TIME
30 to 35 minutes

Baked Artichokes

**10 young artichokes
(see tip)**

fleur de sel

Preheat the oven to 350°F (180°C).

Place the artichokes on a sturdy work surface. Take the artichoke stem in one hand and cut off the top half of the artichoke. If it's there, scrape out the hairy choke at the center of the leaves with a small spoon. Turn the artichoke around and cut the stem off. Remove the hard leaves at the bottom until only soft leaves remain. Place the artichokes in a pot and add enough water to cover; add a little olive oil and season with salt and pepper. Bring to a boil. Cook for 15 to 20 minutes, until a leaf can be easily pulled out.

Drain the artichokes and place them upright in a baking dish. Drizzle with olive oil and season with salt and pepper.

Bake for about 15 minutes until the bottoms of the artichokes are fork-tender, then serve.

TIP: Artichokes

The artichoke is a delicious, beautiful vegetable; it is actually a big flower bud of the thistle family. If you allow artichokes to grow, they will produce gorgeous flowers. The choke turns into pretty purple strings. Young artichokes usually don't have a choke yet, which makes them easier to handle.

Artichokes are excellent for your health. They contain cynarine, a detoxifying substance; additionally, they are a source of prebiotics that are excellent for people with gastrointestinal problems. Prebiotics can be considered food for your intestinal bacteria.

*These artichokes, with a soft, melting
interior and crunchy exterior leaves, are
a gorgeous accompaniment to any meal.*

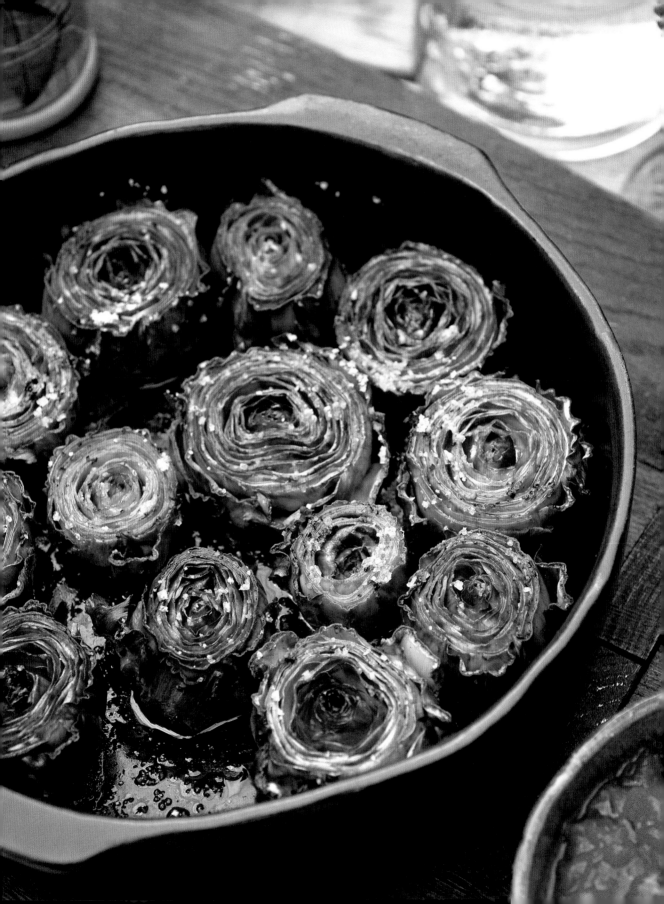

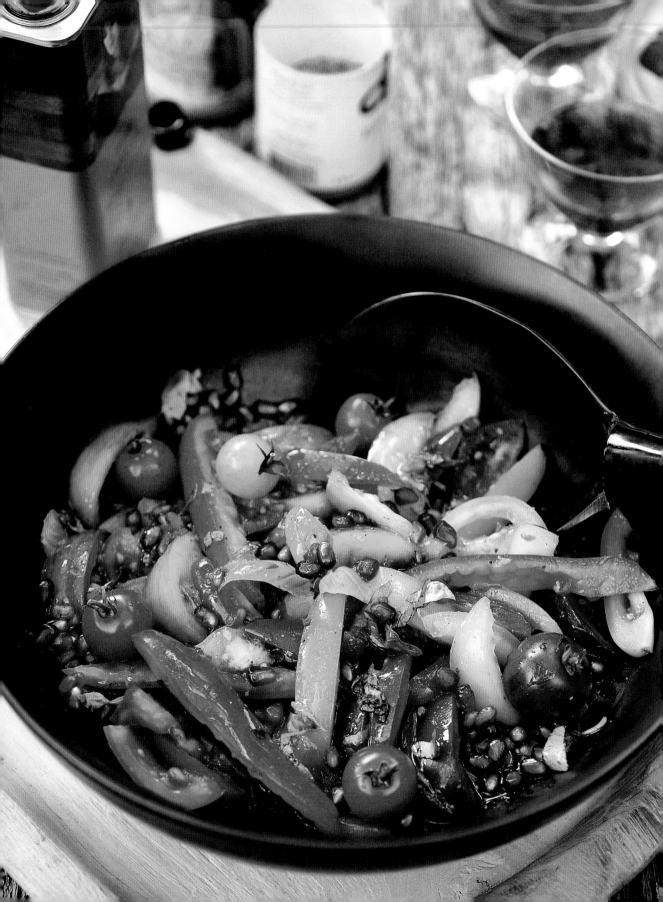

PREPARATION
10 minutes

COOKING TIME
none

Tomato and Pomegranate Medley

various types of
tomatoes (Roma,
yellow, green, orange,
cherry, and so on;
see tip)

1 pomegranate

fleur de sel

Slice the tomatoes into wedges, but leave some of the cherry tomatoes whole. Put them in a serving bowl.

Remove the seeds from the pomegranate (see tip) and toss with the tomatoes. Sprinkle with olive oil and season with pepper and a little fleur de sel.

TIP: Tomatoes
Choose as many different types of tomatoes as you can find: different in shape, color, size, and so on. It is very important that they are all ripe and tender. This way, you get a tomato flavor explosion.

TIP: Pomegranate
Nothing is easier than knocking the seeds out of a pomegranate! Roll the pomegranate on your work surface, pushing down hard with the flat of your palm. You will hear the seeds come loose. Slice the pomegranate in two. Then hold a pomegranate half cut side down over a bowl and beat the skin side of the fruit with a wooden spoon. The seeds will pop right into the bowl.

TIP: Quantity
This is not a meal by itself, but rather a starter or side dish. I decided not to give any quantities for this simple dish. But I would say, eat as much as you like, because it is tasty and healthy.

I always make this during the height of summer, when tomatoes are too plentiful and delicious not to celebrate.

Savoy Cabbage Chips

outer leaves of 1 head savoy cabbage (see tip)

fleur de sel

Preheat the oven to 350°F (180°C).

Pull off the outer leaves of the cabbage (reserve the inner portion of the cabbage for another use). Cut out and discard the thick center ribs of the leaves. Put the leaves in a bowl, add a generous splash of olive oil, and season with fleur de sel and pepper.

Arrange the leaves in a single layer on a baking sheet and bake for 7 minutes, turning the leaves over after 4 or 5 minutes, until crisp.

Check them often! You don't want them to burn (see tip).

TIP: Savoy cabbage
These chips can only be made with the thicker outer leaves of the cabbage—the ones that you would normally discard. Rinse them and pat dry before use.

TIP: 7 minutes at 350°F (180°C)
Every oven is different: I use a convection oven, which usually reduces cooking times. Check often! It is always better to bake for a little while longer at a lower temperature.

This crispy snack is good for you, delicious, and unbelievably beautiful.

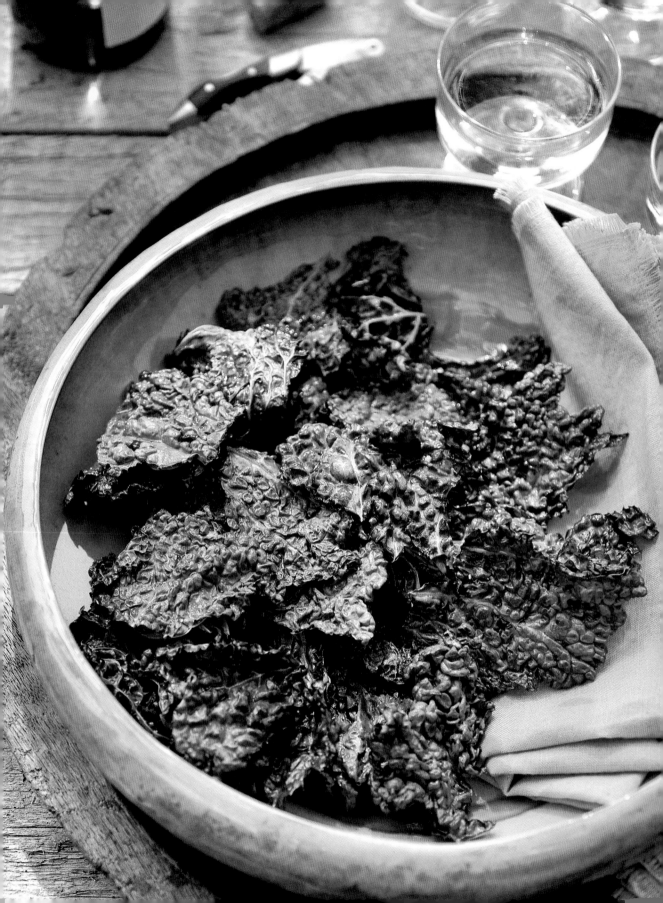

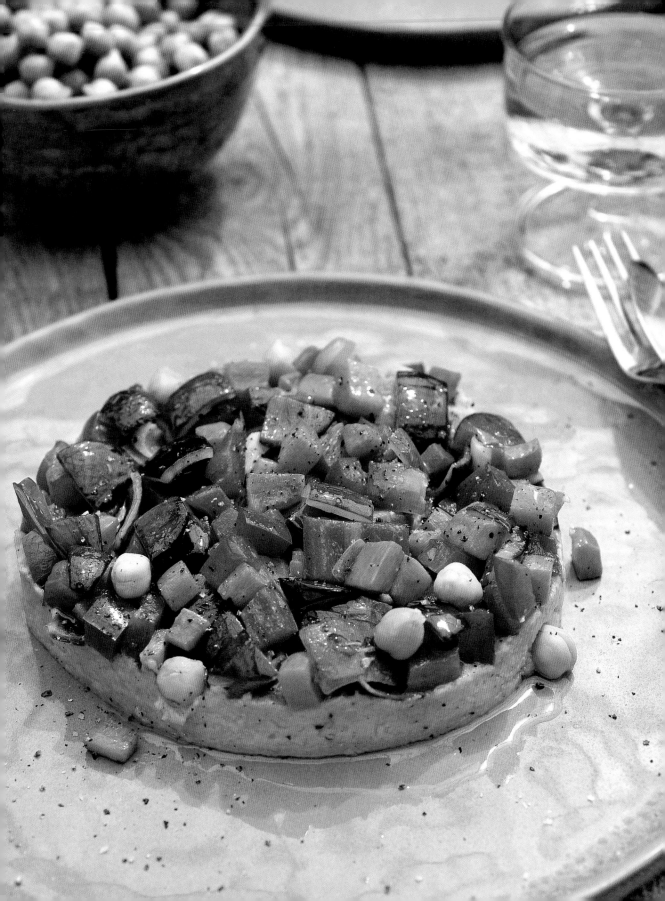

Chickpeas with Carrots, Onions, and Peppers

2 carrots

1 red onion

½ red bell pepper

1 garlic clove

1 (14-ounce/400-g) can chickpeas, drained

1 teaspoon ground cumin

Peel the carrots and dice them, along with the onion and bell pepper.

Heat a splash of olive oil and a little water in a skillet over medium heat. Add the carrots and cook for a few minutes, then add the onion; cook briefly, then add the bell pepper. Cook until softened. If the water evaporates, stir frequently to avoid burning. Season with salt and black pepper.

Mince the garlic and transfer to a food processor. Add the chickpeas, reserving a few for garnish, the cumin, salt, black pepper, and a generous splash of olive oil. Process until the mixture is a thick puree. Transfer to a saucepan and set over low heat.

Take a large ring mold (see tip). Pour the puree into the ring; arrange the vegetables on top and garnish with a few of the reserved chickpeas. Finish with a little olive oil, salt, and black pepper.

TIP: Ring mold

If you don't have a ring mold, you can also simply spoon the puree onto a plate and arrange the vegetables on or around it to make a nice, more free-form presentation.

This colorful combination of vegetables and creamy chickpeas makes for a lovely and filling meal.

SERVES
2

SOAKING TIME
6 hours minimum

PREPARATION
20 minutes

COOKING TIME
15 minutes or so

Savory Lentil and Rice Crêpes with Fresh Herbs

heaping ½ cup (100 g) brown rice

½ cup (100 g) green lentils

2 garlic cloves

3 scallions

2 cups (60 g) stemmed fresh herbs (parsley, arugula, basil, and so on)

Put the rice and lentils in a bowl; cover with water and soak for 6 hours or overnight.

Drain and rinse the lentils and rice. Put them in a food processor with the garlic, scallions, and salt and pepper. Add some water and process until you obtain a thick, smooth batter. If the batter is too thick, add more water and keep on processing until the mixture has the consistency of pancake batter.

Finely chop the herbs and toss them with salt, pepper, and olive oil.

Heat a small nonstick sauté pan over medium-high heat. Drizzle the pan with olive oil and tilt the pan to coat. Ladle in about ¼ cup (60 ml) of the batter (depending on the size of your pan) and spread it with a spatula to coat the surface of the pan. Cook until the batter looks dry and the edges are slightly browned, and the crêpes are not sticking to the pan, then flip and cook the other side. Transfer to a plate and repeat with the remaining batter, using more olive oil as necessary to keep the crêpes from sticking. While cooking, stack the crêpes and keep them in a warm place.

Spread herbs over each crêpe and roll or fold shut. Serve immediately.

TIP: Dosa
This recipe is inspired by the traditional Indian pancakes called dosa. Dosa are often eaten for breakfast or as a snack. They are stuffed with all sorts of vegetables: sautéed onions, seasoned potatoes, and so on. They are wonderfully crunchy and full of flavor. I have created my own version with fresh herbs. Remember to mix the batter long enough to eliminate lumps. You can also make very thin crêpes if you strain the batter.

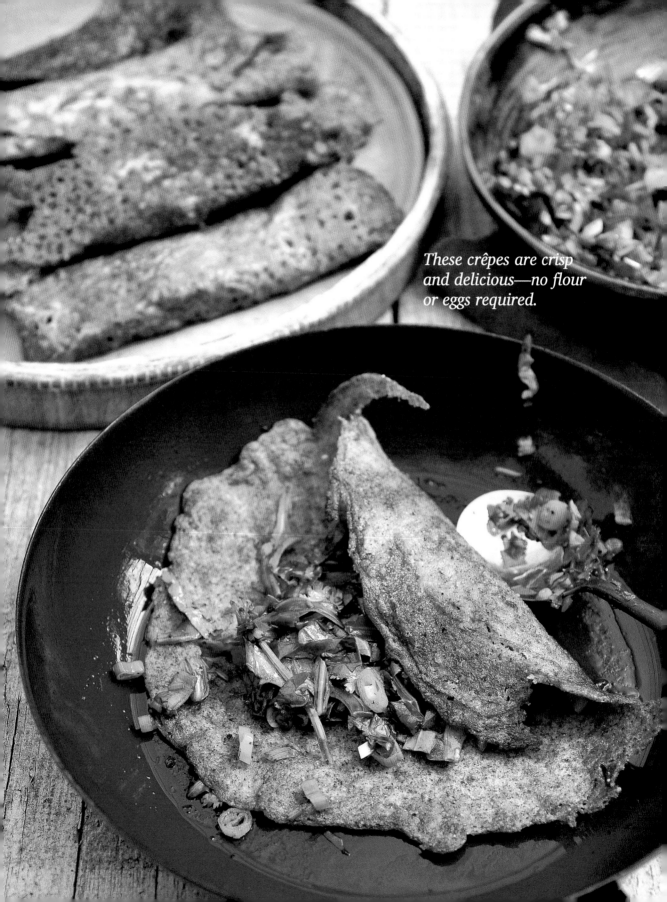

These crêpes are crisp and delicious—no flour or eggs required.

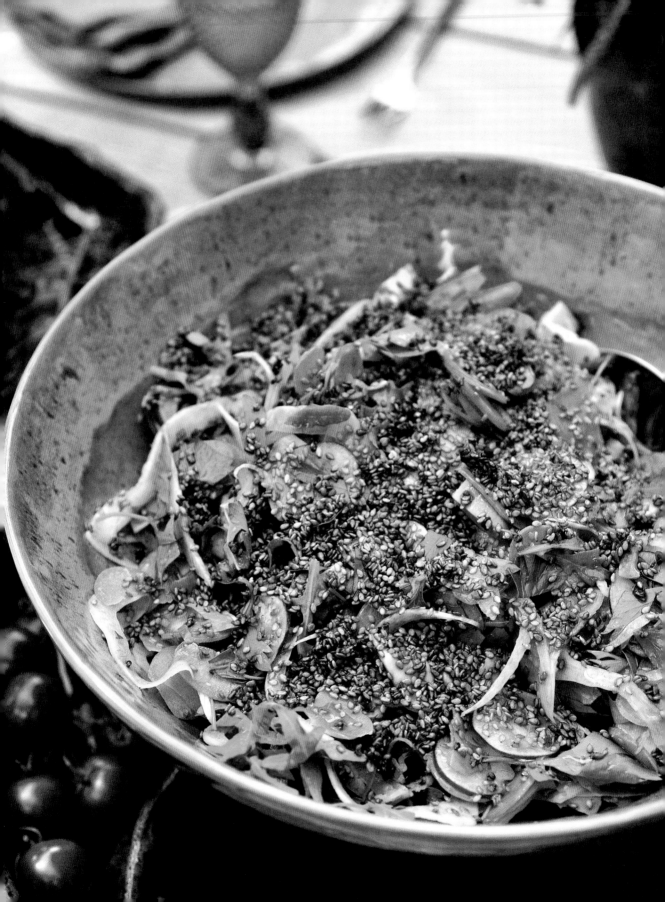

SERVES
2

PREPARATION
20 minutes

MARINATING
15 minutes minimum

COOKING TIME
6 to 10 minutes

Avocado, Fennel, Carrot, and Radish Salad with Marinated Sesame Seeds

sesame seeds (natural or toasted) (see tips, page 135)

soy sauce

1 bulb fennel

2 carrots

1 bunch radishes

1 avocado

arugula or other fresh herbs

Preheat the oven to 350°F (180°C). Line a baking sheet with parchment paper.

Put the sesame seeds in a small bowl and add enough soy sauce to cover them. Let sit for at least 15 minutes, or until the soy sauce has been almost totally absorbed.

Spread the marinated sesame seeds over the prepared baking sheet. Bake for 6 to 10 minutes. Check the seeds frequently to avoid burning; they should dry evenly and become crispy. They should not become dark brown; take them out when they are lightly browned. If necessary, lower the oven temperature and let them roast a little longer.

Peel the carrots and slice them, along with the radishes and fennel, as thinly as possible. This is best done with a mandoline. (A peeler also works well for the carrots, but not for radishes and fennel. Of course, you can also slice them by hand.) Pit, peel, and dice the avocado. Combine the sliced vegetables, avocado, arugula, and a generous splash of olive oil in a bowl, season with pepper only (the sesame seeds are already salty), and toss gently.

Sprinkle with the sesame seeds and serve.

The flavorful crunch from the sesame seeds takes this salad to the next level.

Wild Rice Salad with Fennel and Herbs

1¼ cups (215 g) wild rice (see tip)

1 bunch cilantro

2 scallions

1 bulb fennel

For the dressing:

2 to 3 tablespoons salted shelled peanuts

5 tablespoons toasted sesame oil

2 garlic cloves

1 (½-inch/12-mm) piece fresh ginger

juice of 1 lime

Rinse the rice and cook it in water according to the package directions (usually 45 minutes to 1 hour). Drain if necessary and set aside to let it cool.

Finely chop the cilantro and scallions and thinly slice the fennel.

Make the dressing: Coarsely chop the peanuts and mix them with the sesame oil. Mince the garlic and ginger and add to the peanuts; add the lime juice.

Toss the wild rice together with the cilantro, scallions, fennel, and sauce and serve the salad in a pretty bowl.

TIP: Wild rice

Wild rice is actually not rice—it is the seed of a grasslike aquatic plant that is related to rice. The seeds have a delicious nutty flavor and are dark brown to black, which makes them particularly attractive to cooks who play with colors in the kitchen. They burst open when cooked. Name aside, the "wild" rice in supermarkets is usually cultivated, but the seeds are whole and unrefined, making them as nutritious and healthy as the true wild variety.

TIP: Fennel

Fennel discolors quickly; sprinkle it with a few drops of lime juice immediately after cutting to prevent this.

Chewy rice with a delicious nutty flavor and a lime-ginger dressing . . . I love this tart, hearty salad!

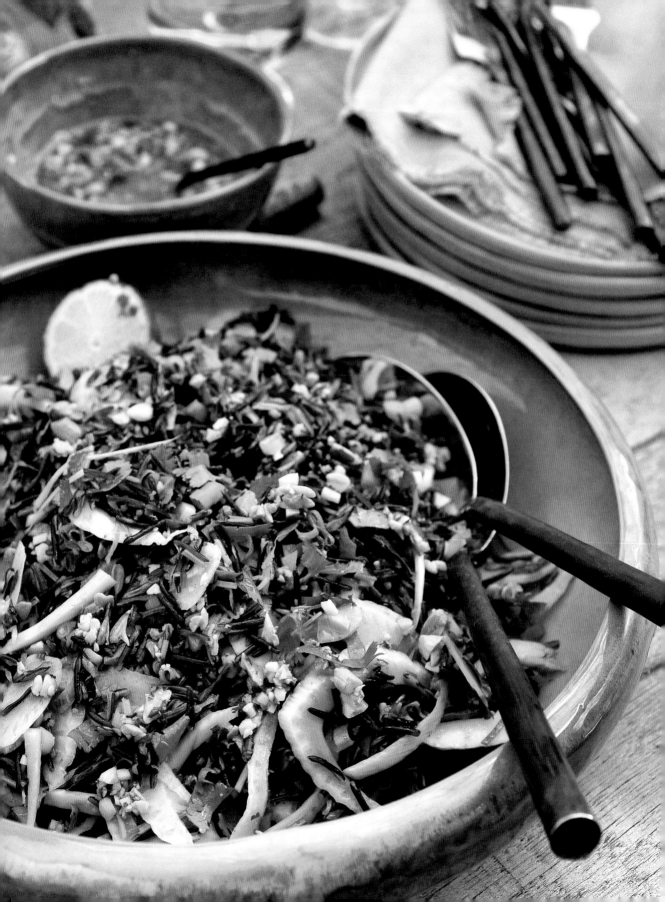

Good Bacteria and Nutrition

DON'T IGNORE YOUR GUT.

Telling someone they are smart is one of the nicest compliments you can give. That is because anything that has to do with "brains" is highly regarded. However, gut feelings or instincts don't get as much praise—especially because a gut feeling originates in our intestines. Just the word *guts* makes many people uncomfortable.

Intestines are one of the most exciting research areas of current biology. Practically every emotion can be felt in your belly, like butterflies or a knot in your stomach. We can feel these sensations because our intestines include a network of neurons. Since this network is so developed and can operate independently from our brain, some scientists have even given it the nickname "our second brain."[10]

The intestinal nervous system is equipped with its own reflexes and senses; this makes it the largest sensory organ in our body. The intestinal nervous system operates independently and is not controlled by the brain. According to American intestine specialist Michael Gershon—a pioneer in this area and author of the book *The Second Brain*—our emotions are actually influenced by nerves in our intestines. He demonstrated that the information channel from the intestines to the brain is at least as important as that from the brain to the intestines.

New studies are focusing on our intestinal flora and the importance of bacteria throughout the course of our lives. Before birth, we are free of microbes; as soon as we pass through the birth canal, we absorb our mother's bacteria. These are very important for the microbe mass that we build. The following years are crucial. We continuously take in bacteria through contact with our environment. Whether we grow up in a city or in the country, the type of food we eat, the hands we shake, the people we live with, the experiences we have during our foreign travels, and so on—all of these circumstances impact our bacterial load, what we now call the microbiota, the microbes that live in us.

People once believed that bacteria only caused problems and should thus be eliminated. However, the consensus now is that most bacteria are harmless and play a key role in our health. They help us with all sorts of tasks that we could not perform otherwise. Bacteria train our immune system; they protect us from other pathogenic bacteria, from fungi and viruses; they break down toxins; they help us process indigestible food; they provide energy to our intestines; and they produce vitamins and other substances that our body needs to function properly.

[10] One of them is Michael Gershon, director of the Department of Anatomy and Cell Biology of the New York Presbyterian Hospital/ Columbia University Medical Center, an expert in neurogastroenterology and author of *The Second Brain* (HarperCollins, 1998).

"As a professor, I am always a skeptic; however, I believe that our intestinal bacteria have an impact on what happens in our brain," says Dr. Emeran Mayer.[11] Mayer compared the brain structure of volunteers with their individual type of intestinal bacteria in order to demonstrate such connections.

In 2013, UCLA researchers presented evidence that bacteria can impact brain functions through nutrition. For four weeks, healthy women received a mixture of specific bacteria twice a day. Researchers were surprised to see the effects on the brain. This suggests that we could improve brain functions through nutrition, says Dr. Kirsten Tillisch.[12]

There is indeed still a lot to discover; however, there is undoubtedly a connection between nutrition, the bacteria in our intestines, and our brain. It appears from a multitude of studies that there is a connection between a disturbed intestinal flora and certain diseases: obesity, diabetes, some cancers, Crohn's disease, celiac disease, asthma, autism, and so on. Consequently, it is in our best interest to keep our intestinal flora healthy. Somebody with an extensive supply of good bacteria is better protected against all sorts of diseases. Biodiversity is not only important in nature: It is also crucial in your intestines.

HOW CAN WE TAKE GOOD CARE OF OUR INTESTINAL FLORA?
First, scientists insist on the fact that we should be cautious about using antibiotics because they also kill good bacteria. Second, nutrition plays an important role in influencing intestinal bacteria. We can stimulate the diversity of our microbiota by eating varied and, most important, natural, unprocessed, and fiber-rich foods. This type of food has evolved for millions of years, as have the bacteria in our belly.

It has become increasingly clear to me over the years how important it is to eat natural foods. In nature, everything is nicely balanced. Take something out of a natural chain, and you instantly cause problems. This delicate balance with the environment also applies to humans. We are connected to our environment, we are not alone: The hundred trillion bacteria in our gut determine how we feel and how we behave.[13] Just as we are connected to the world, these bacteria are also connected to us. How we live in harmony will determine our level of health.

---

[11] Dr. Emeran Mayer is a professor of medicine and psychiatry at UCLA.

[12] Kirsten Tillisch et al., "Consumption of Fermented Milk Product with Probiotic Modulates Brain Activity," *Gastroenterology* 144, no. 7 (June 2013): 1394–1401. Kirsten Tillisch is affiliated with UCLA: https://www.uclahealth.org/.

[13] An absolute must-read on the intestinal function is the book *Gut: The Inside Story of Our Body's Most Underrated Organ*, by young German author Giulia Enders.

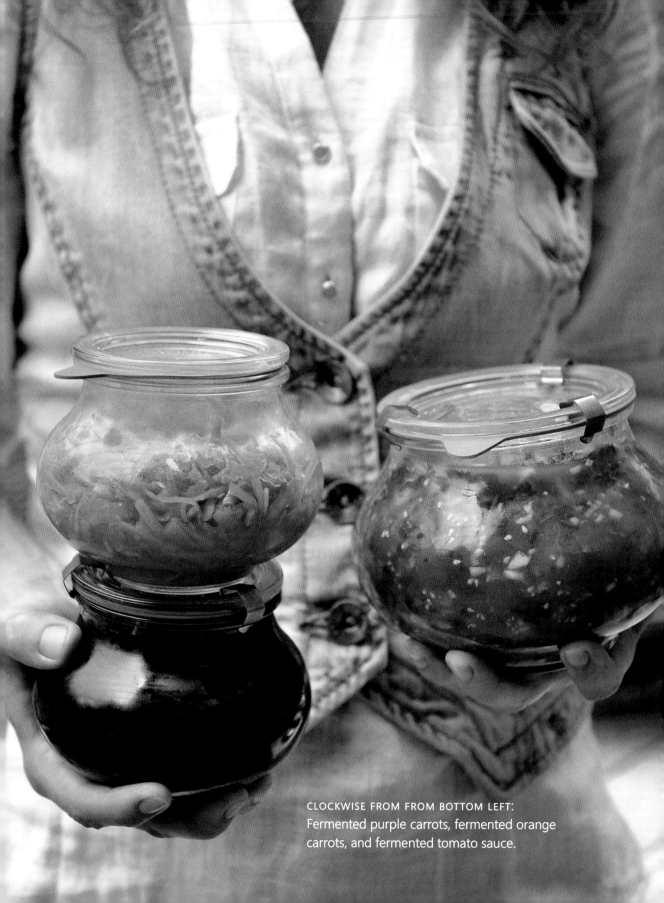

CLOCKWISE FROM FROM BOTTOM LEFT:
Fermented purple carrots, fermented orange carrots, and fermented tomato sauce.

Fermented Vegetables

WHAT IS FERMENTING?

Fermenting is one of the oldest food preservation methods. Today, it is back in vogue, not so much to preserve food—because nothing beats the safety of a refrigerator or freezer—but because of the healthy bacteria that are created during fermentation. With this process, healthy bacteria have the opportunity to grow abundantly, and bad bacteria, fungi, and yeasts are eliminated. Vegetable fermentation requires an oxygen-free environment. Therefore, you must seal the vegetables in jars topped with a bag of water (called a water seal). Warmth and moisture allow microorganisms to grow, producing enzymes that break off specific nutrients (such as carbohydrates and protein), thereby changing the taste, smell, and digestibility of the product.

WHY ARE FERMENTED PRODUCTS HEALTHY?

– They contain good bacteria that stimulate our intestinal flora and digestion.
– They are more nutritious than the original ingredient, because the nutrients are easier to digest, thus better absorbed into our bodies.
– They contain high concentrations of vitamins, primarily B, C, and K.
– They strengthen the intestinal wall, which in turn boosts our immune system.

WHAT IS THE DIFFERENCE BETWEEN PROBIOTICS AND PREBIOTICS?

Probiotics are living microorganisms or, simply put, healthy bacteria. Fermentation stimulates and multiplies them. Bacteria primarily live in your large intestine. Our enzymes cannot digest some nutrients, such as specific fibers and sugars. They stay undigested in the large intestine, where they serve as food for the good bacteria. They help make our gut healthy and strong. The gut is one of the most important organs for our health. Fermented food is a rich source of probiotics. Along with the dishes on pages 180 and 181, sauerkraut, yogurt, and kefir also have high contents of probiotics; however, in most cases, such products are pasteurized, a process that destroys a lot of valuable bacteria. Asian cuisines have the richest traditions of fermented foods, such as miso, soy sauce, tempeh (fermented soybeans), and kimchi (spicy fermented cabbage).

Prebiotics are food for these healthy bacteria. Rich natural sources of prebiotics are artichokes, legumes, garlic, salsify, onions, asparagus, chicory, endive, oatmeal (cooked and cooled), potatoes, apples, and berries.

Ideally, combine probiotics and prebiotics in your diet—this is called synbiotics.

MAKES
about 3½ cups (400 g)

PREPARATION
20 minutes

COOKING TIME
3 days

Fermented Carrots

14 ounces (400 g) carrots

½ cup (40 g) peeled and sliced ginger

1 teaspoon fleur de sel (do not use ordinary kitchen salt)

1 (64-ounce/2-liter) sterilized glass jar

1 (32-ounce/1-liter) sterilized glass jar

a plastic zip-top freezer bag

bottled water

Cut the carrots lengthwise into ribbons with a peeler. Peel and mince the ginger. Toss the carrots and ginger in a bowl with the fleur de sel. Wash your hands thoroughly and begin kneading until the carrots release their juices (carrots don't have a lot).

Put the mixture in the large jar. Make a fist and firmly push the carrots downward until the jar is about half-filled. Carrots release only small amounts of juice; therefore, add a little bottled still water (not tap water). Don't add too much: only enough to cover the carrots. Place a plastic zip-top freezer bag inside the jar and fill it with water (for this, you can use tap water). Seal the bag. The weight of the bag will keep the carrots submerged in the brine (this is called a "water seal"). Place a couple of kitchen towels over the jar and set aside at room temperature for 3 days.

After 3 days, remove the towels and the water seal. You should see small bubbles around the rim: This is normal; it is the fermentation in process. Transfer the carrots to the smaller jar; fill it to the rim. Seal the jar tightly with a lid and store the carrots in the refrigerator. This will keep for a few months.

TIP: Fermentation
Fermentation may be somewhat intimidating. You will find a lot of information on the subject on the Internet (YouTube, for example) with videos that will be very helpful. Many people are worried about doing something wrong; however, it is really not difficult. Just try it!

TIP: Hygiene is important
Fermentation is nothing other than a controlled spoilage process. In this process, we only want the good bacteria; therefore, it is important to always work in a very clean environment and with thoroughly washed containers. Run them through the dishwasher on the hot cycle, or wash by hand with hot, soapy water and rinse well.

MAKES
about 2 cups (500 g)

PREPARATION
20 minutes

COOKING TIME
3 days

Fermented Tomato Sauce

18 ounces (500 g) cherry tomatoes

2 shallots

2 garlic cloves

1 bunch cilantro

juice of ½ lime

1 teaspoon fleur de sel (do not use ordinary kitchen salt)

1 (64-ounce/2-liter) sterilized glass jar

1 (32-ounce/1-liter) sterilized glass jar

a plastic zip-top freezer bag

Cut the tomatoes into quarters and chop the shallots, garlic, and cilantro. Combine all in a bowl; add the lime juice and fleur de sel.

Wash your hands thoroughly and knead the mixture until the vegetables release their juices. This will take 3 to 5 minutes.

Pour the mixture into the large jar. It will probably be only half-full, and that is exactly what we need. Make a fist and push the vegetables down to remove all air bubbles. Place a plastic zip-top freezer bag inside the jar and fill it with water (tap water is fine for this). Seal the bag. Place a couple of kitchen towels over the jar and set aside at room temperature for 3 days.

Transfer the fermented tomatoes to the smaller jar; fill it to the rim so that very little air can penetrate.

Close the jar tightly with a lid and store in the refrigerator. The (closed) jar can be kept for a couple of months.

TIP: Good reads

If you would like to learn more about fermentation, I recommend *The Art of Fermentation*, by Sandor Ellix Katz (Chelsea Green Publishing, 2012).

An absolute must-read on the intestinal function is *Gut: The Inside Story of Our Body's Most Underrated Organ* (Greystone Books, 2015), by the young German author Giulia Enders. Everyone should read this book to gain insight and respect for the wonderful, ingenious work of our guts. Even though it is a scientifically based book, it is very readable and written with great humor.

Fermented products have an acidic flavor similar to pickles. After you have become accustomed to these umami-laden treats, you will love them. I usually serve fermented foods with salads or dishes with meat or fish.

My Delicious Fruit Breakfast

Every one of my cookbooks includes a recipe for a fruit breakfast, because fruits, along with vegetables, form the basis of my healthy cooking.

The best thing I have ever done is to replace bread with fruit, and potatoes with other, more nutritious vegetables.

Not only have these changes freed me from my addiction to fast carbohydrates, but also it was the beginning of a new life, full of energy and without weight issues. You feel that this natural food has much more to offer your body in all areas: pleasure, health, and freedom. Well-known research professor Richard Béliveau, who specializes in cancer research, calls fruit and vegetables "the best anti-cancer diet." Dr. Oyinlola Oyebode of University College London, head of a large-scale study in England, concluded: "It is clear that the more vegetables and fruit you eat, the less chance you have to die of cancer or heart problems, regardless of your age."[14]

Contrary to what many believe, fresh fruits are not fast carbohydrates. That's because while fruits contain sugars, they also provide a lot of fiber, water, and many health-promoting plant compounds, which cause the sugar in the fruit to be released slowly. It is important to eat the entire fruit, preferably with skin if it is edible. Fruit and fruit juice smoothies are not a good idea because they break apart or eliminate the fibers; consequently, sugars are released faster. It is not true that by eating fruit you consume too much sugar.

I used to be an avid bread eater; I just couldn't stop. I'd often have toast for breakfast, but bread, even whole wheat, is rich in carbohydrates.

Now, I can't do without my fruit breakfast. It is unbelievably tasty and very filling; you cannot eat too much of it. With every bite, you know you are consuming a large variety of vitamins, minerals, and other nutrients that strengthen your body. No need to count calories; just enjoy the colors, flavors, and juicy textures that nature offers us. This is pleasure and freedom. I like to add mixed seeds and coconut milk or yogurt. This makes for a well-balanced, nutritious, and satisfying start to your day.

[14] Dr. Oyinlola Oyebode, Department of Epidemiology and Public Health, UCL.

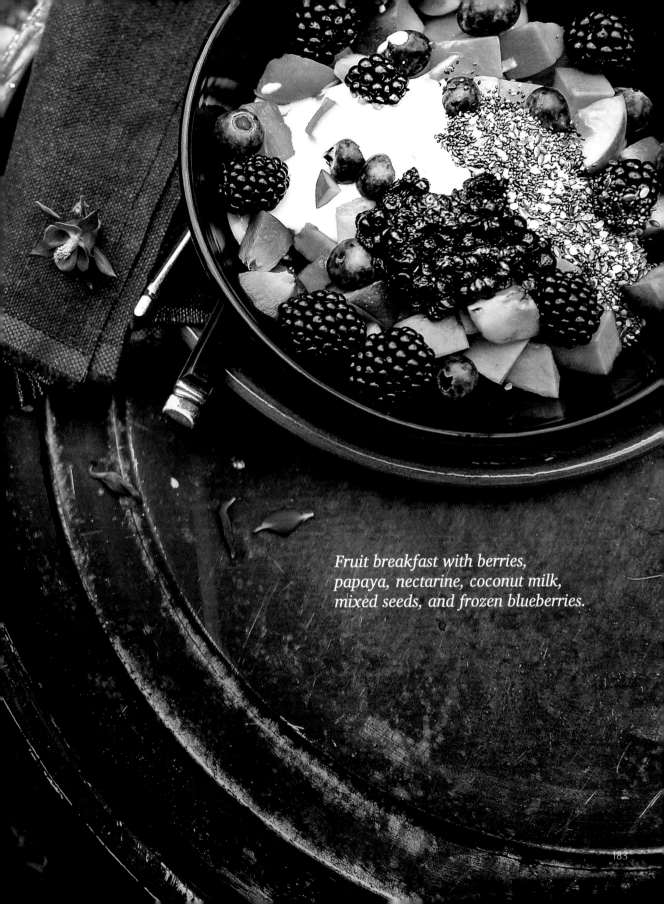

*Fruit breakfast with berries,
papaya, nectarine, coconut milk,
mixed seeds, and frozen blueberries.*

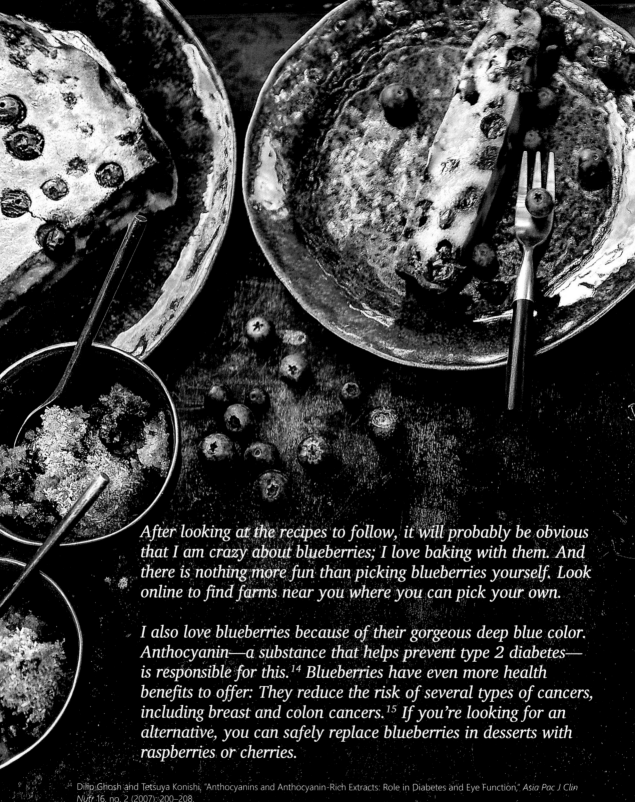

After looking at the recipes to follow, it will probably be obvious that I am crazy about blueberries; I love baking with them. And there is nothing more fun than picking blueberries yourself. Look online to find farms near you where you can pick your own.

I also love blueberries because of their gorgeous deep blue color. Anthocyanin—a substance that helps prevent type 2 diabetes— is responsible for this.[14] Blueberries have even more health benefits to offer: They reduce the risk of several types of cancers, including breast and colon cancers.[15] If you're looking for an alternative, you can safely replace blueberries in desserts with raspberries or cherries.

[14] Dilip Ghosh and Tetsuya Konishi, "Anthocyanins and Anthocyanin-Rich Extracts: Role in Diabetes and Eye Function," *Asia Pac J Clin Nutr* 16, no. 2 (2007): 200–208.

[15] Richard Béliveau and Denis Gingras, *Foods That Fight Cancer: Preventing Cancer Through Diet* (Toronto: McClelland & Stewart, 2005).

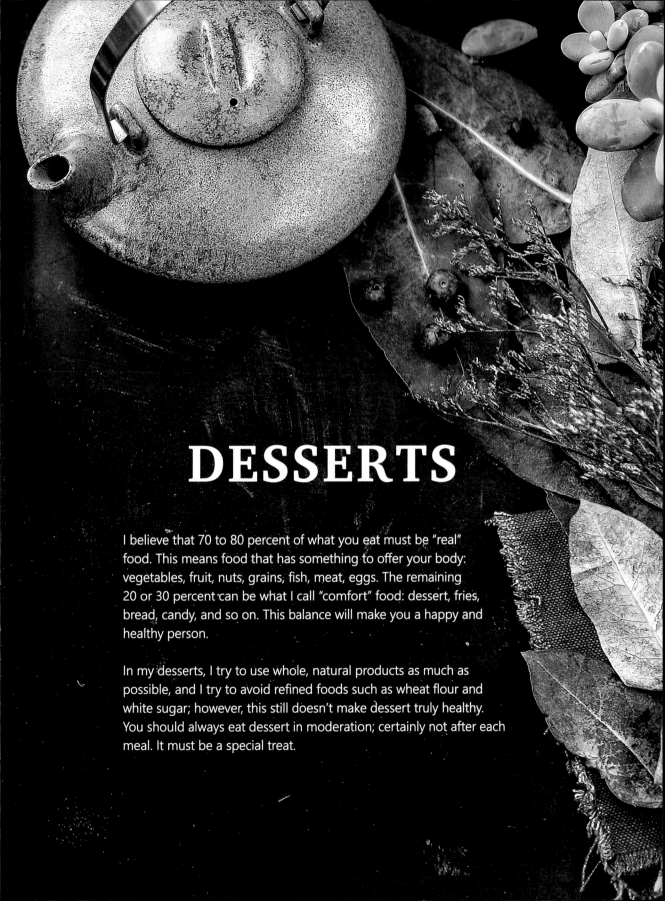

DESSERTS

I believe that 70 to 80 percent of what you eat must be "real" food. This means food that has something to offer your body: vegetables, fruit, nuts, grains, fish, meat, eggs. The remaining 20 or 30 percent can be what I call "comfort" food: dessert, fries, bread, candy, and so on. This balance will make you a happy and healthy person.

In my desserts, I try to use whole, natural products as much as possible, and I try to avoid refined foods such as wheat flour and white sugar; however, this still doesn't make dessert truly healthy. You should always eat dessert in moderation; certainly not after each meal. It must be a special treat.

MAKES
1 (9½ by 6½-inch/24 by
16-cm) cake

PREPARATION
10 minutes

COOKING TIME
20 to 30 minutes

Fluffy Blueberry Cake

¼ cup (55 g) good-quality butter

2 eggs

⅓ cup (60 g) coconut sugar (see tip)

1 scant cup (100 g) almond flour (see tip)

6 tablespoons (90 ml) whole-milk yogurt (or full-fat coconut milk) (see tip)

7 ounces (200 g) fresh blueberries

Preheat the oven to 350°F (180°C). Grease a 9½ by 6½-inch (24 by 16-cm) baking dish (see tip).

Melt the butter and set aside to cool.

In a bowl, mix the eggs, coconut sugar, almond flour, and yogurt; stir in the cooled melted butter. Gently fold in the blueberries. Pour the mixture into the prepared baking dish and bake for 20 minutes, or until the surface is dry but the inside is still a bit moist. Let cool for a few minutes before serving.

TIP: Coconut sugar

I like to use coconut sugar, primarily because of its flavor: It adds a delicious caramel taste to all your desserts. It is an unrefined sugar, and some studies show that it might not increase your blood sugar as much as regular sugar, although this is controversial. If you can't find coconut sugar, you can use grated palm sugar, honey, agave, or maple syrup. So, can we consider any of these healthy sugars? No, I don't think that exists. Therefore, I use a little sugar just every once in a while.

TIP: Almond flour

Almond flour can be found in most grocery stores and natural foods stores; however, it is also easy to make it at home. Buy 3 ounces (80 g) raw almonds and process them in a blender or food processor until you have flour. That's it.

TIP: Yogurt

It is important to use natural full-fat yogurt. If you use skimmed yogurt, your cake will fall apart. It is the fat that binds.

TIP: Baking dish

I make my own ceramics and oven dishes and I like to use one of these as a baking mold. If using a ceramic dish, I use parchment paper to prevent sticking. Using a beautiful oven dish means that you can just serve the cake straight from the pan.

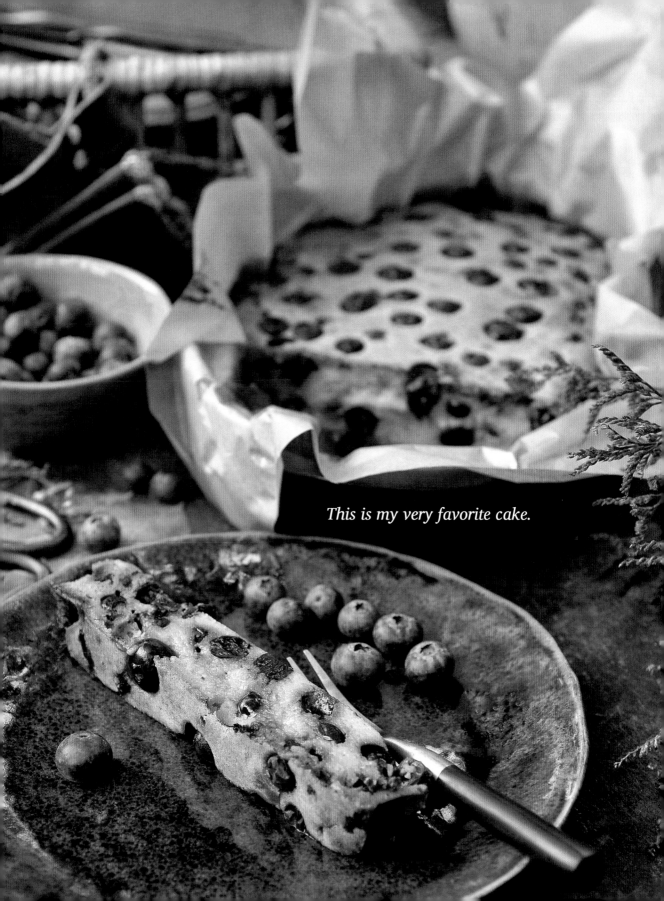

This is my very favorite cake.

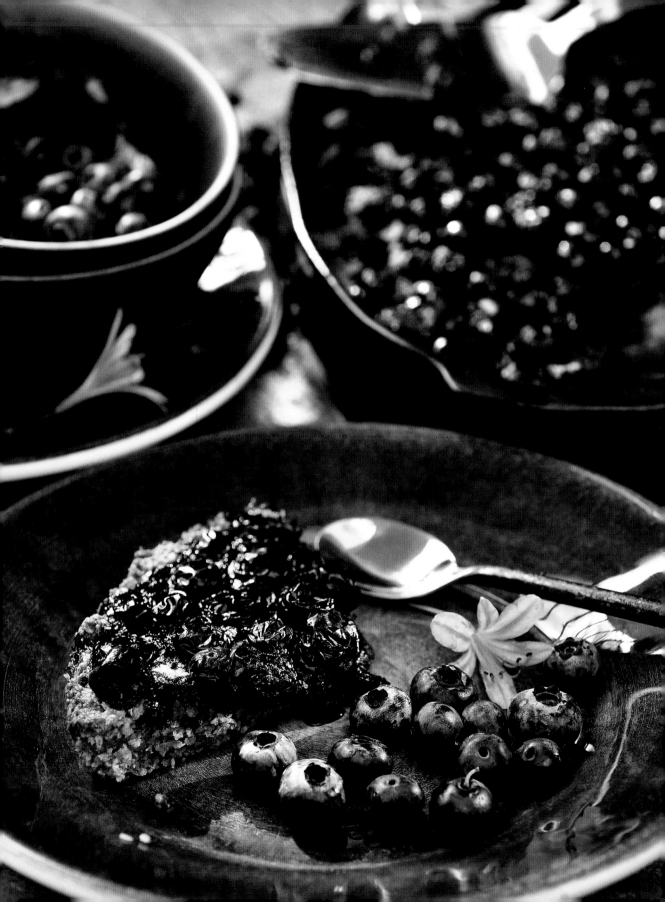

MAKES
1 (8-inch/20-cm) round
dessert

PREPARATION
10 minutes

COOKING TIME
30 minutes

Blueberry Crumble Tart

2 cups (200 g) oat
bran

7 ounces (200 g)
good-quality butter

¼ cup (40 g) coconut
sugar (see tip, page
186)

1 egg

7 ounces (200 g)
blueberries

Preheat the oven to 350°F (180°C). Line an 8-inch (20-cm) round baking pan with parchment paper (both the bottom and sides of the pan should be covered).

In a bowl, mix the oat bran, butter, coconut sugar, and egg. It is actually fun to mix with your hands. Knead vigorously until you can roll the dough into a ball. Place the dough in the prepared pan and press it into a flat disk with the edges a little higher than the center. Sprinkle the berries over the center and gently push them into the dough. Bake for 20 to 30 minutes until crust is golden brown. Let cool before slicing.

TIP: Bran
Bran is the sheath of the grain, and the healthiest part because it contains the most fiber, vitamins, and minerals. You can buy oat bran at natural food stores.

A rich, crunchy blueberry dessert that you can easily slice to take along with you on picnics and trips.

MAKES
1 (8-inch/20-cm) round
dessert

PREPARATION
10 minutes

COOKING TIME
20 minutes

Shredded Coconut Crumble

6 tablespoons (85 g) good-quality butter

1 cup plus 3 tablespoons (100 g) shredded unsweetened coconut

⅓ cup (60 g) coconut sugar (see tip, page 186)

2 eggs

7 ounces (200 g) blueberries

Preheat the oven to 350°F (180°C).

Melt the butter and set aside to cool slightly.

In a bowl, mix 1 cup (85 g) of the coconut, the coconut sugar, and eggs. Add the cooled melted butter. Gently fold in the blueberries. Pour the mixture into an 8-inch (20-cm) round baking dish (see tip). Sprinkle with the remaining coconut, and bake for 20 minutes until the top is light brown and a toothpick or knife inserted in the center comes out clean.

This dessert cannot be sliced; the best way to serve it is to place the baking dish on your table and scoop the crumble into small bowls.

TIP: Baking dish
Any ovenproof dish will do, and you don't need to prepare the dish before baking. I usually serve the dessert straight from the baking dish, so I use the ceramics that I design.

I like serving this very satisfying dessert while it is still warm from the oven.

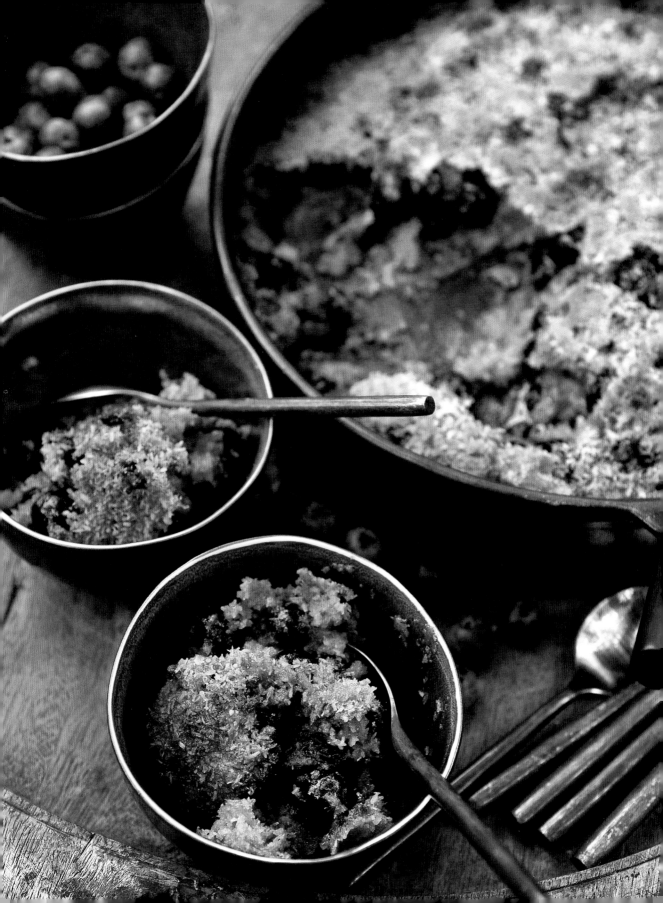

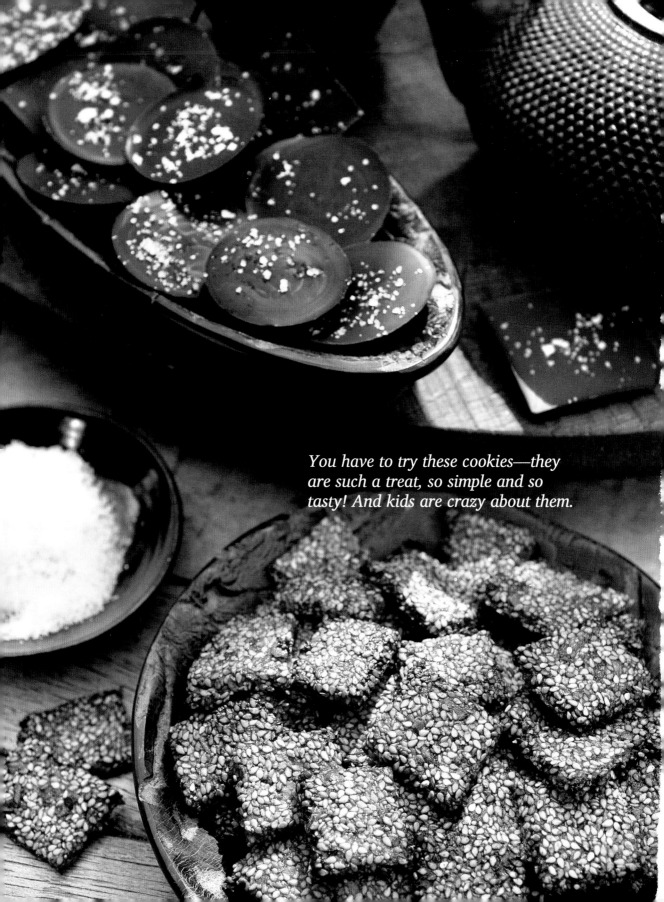

You have to try these cookies—they are such a treat, so simple and so tasty! And kids are crazy about them.

Fleur de Sel Chocolates

MAKES
10 pieces

PREPARATION
5 minutes

COOKING TIME
10 minutes

3½ ounces (100 g) dark chocolate (a minimum of 70% cacao)

pinch fleur de sel

Melt the chocolate in a double boiler or in a bowl set over a saucepan of simmering water (do not let the bottom of the bowl touch the water). Pour the chocolate into small ramekins (or in a muffin tin). Let cool for about 5 minutes, then sprinkle with fleur de sel. Place the ramekins in the refrigerator until the chocolate is completely set. Remove the chocolate from the ramekins and serve.

TIP: Storage

Cover the chocolates with a cloth and store in a cool, dry place. If you keep them in the refrigerator, cover them with plastic wrap.

Crispy Sesame Seed–Fig Cookies

MAKES
about 20 cookies

PREPARATION
10 minutes

COOKING TIME
20 to 30 minutes

1⅓ cups (200 g) dried figs

⅔ cup (100 g) unhulled sesame seeds (see tip)

Preheat the oven to 350°F (180°C). Line a baking sheet with parchment paper.

Stem the figs and place in a food processor. Process to a paste. Transfer the paste to a bowl and knead in the sesame seeds. Press the mixture flat on the prepared baking sheet. To evenly spread the thick paste, place a sheet of parchment paper on top and then a baking dish on top of that and press everything down. The thinner the dough, the crispier the cookies. Make shallow cuts in the dough; this will make it easier to break the cookies apart after baking.

Bake for 10 minutes, then lower the oven temperature to 280°F (140°C) and bake another 10 minutes. If you like your cookies totally crispy, flip the cookies over and bake for 10 minutes more. Make sure they don't burn!

TIP: Unhulled sesame seeds

Sesame seeds are often sold hulled or toasted, but this recipe will be much tastier and healthier if you use unhulled sesame seeds, which are a good source of fiber, calcium, potassium, magnesium, manganese, and selenium.

SERVES
2 to 4

PREPARATION
10 minutes

COOKING TIME
15 to 20 minutes

Baked Peaches with Mascarpone

2 peaches (see tip)

8 ounces (225 g) mascarpone

3 tablespoons honey

handful of slivered almonds

fresh unsprayed lavender flowers (optional)

Preheat the oven to 350°F (180°C).

Halve and pit the peaches. Place them cut side up in a baking dish. Mix the mascarpone and honey, and spoon it over the peaches. Sprinkle with the slivered almonds and bake for 15 to 20 minutes, until the peaches are soft. Garnish with some lavender flowers, if desired.

TIP: Dessert or breakfast?

This is a delicious, filling dish. As a dessert, I would serve half a peach per person; as a breakfast, I would definitely serve one full peach per person.

This is a real treat, whether you serve it as dessert or a special breakfast.

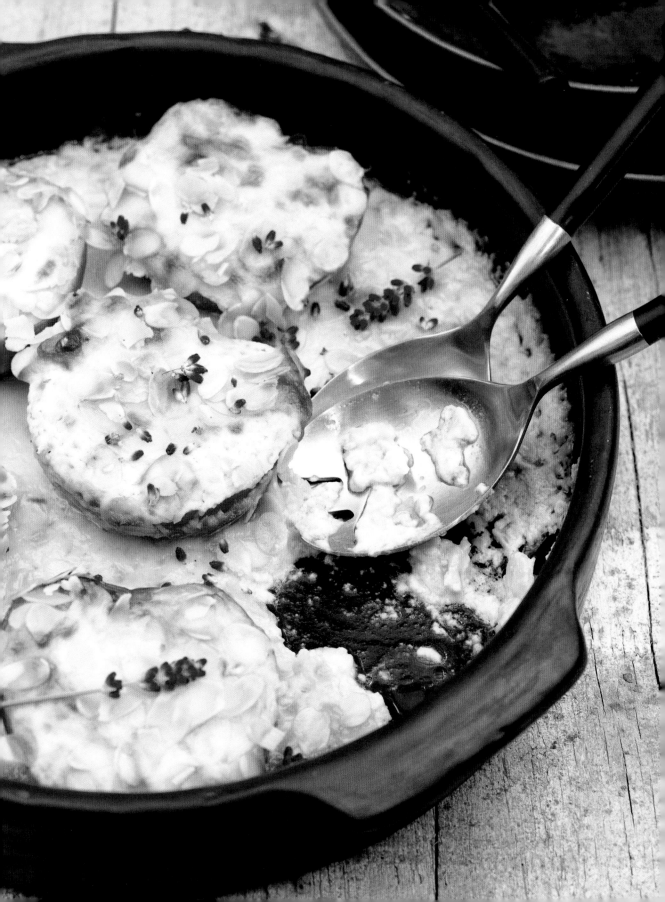

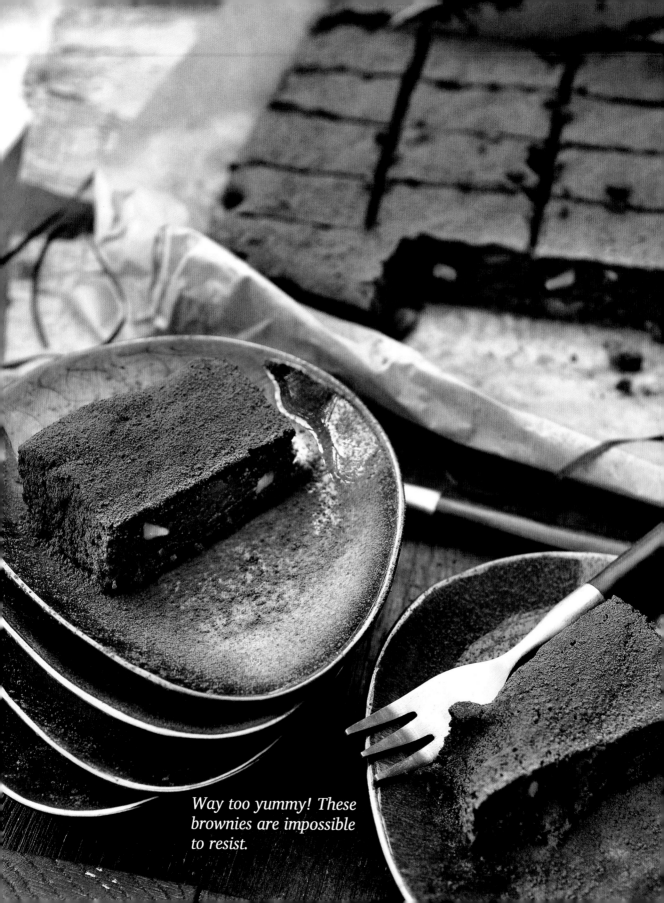

Way too yummy! These brownies are impossible to resist.

MAKES
7 or 8 brownies

PREPARATION
15 minutes

COOKING TIME
20 minutes

Delicious Flourless Brownies

4 ounces (115 g) dark chocolate

7 tablespoons (100 g) good-quality butter

1 heaping cup (150 g) whole almonds

6 dried apricots (see tip)

2 eggs

¼ cup (40 g) coconut sugar (see tip, page 186)

unsweetened cocoa powder (optional)

Preheat the oven to 350°F (180°C). Grease a 6-inch (15-cm) square baking pan or line it with parchment paper.

Break the chocolate into pieces and melt them with the butter in a double boiler or in a heatproof bowl set over a saucepan of simmering water (make sure the water does not touch the bottom of the bowl). Do not overheat the chocolate-butter mixture. Stir until well combined and smooth. Remove from the heat and let cool (see tip).

Grind two-thirds of the almonds in a blender or food processor to obtain a coarse meal (it doesn't have to be as fine as flour). Finely chop the remaining almonds and the apricots by hand.

Whisk the eggs and coconut sugar in a bowl until foamy. With a spoon, stir in the ground almonds and the chopped almonds and apricots. Add the cooled, melted chocolate and stir briefly to combine.

Pour the batter into the prepared baking pan. The batter should be ¾ to 1 inch (2 to 2.5 cm) thick. Bake for 15 minutes until just set in the middle.

If you can wait, let it cool on a wire rack for 15 minutes. If you like soft, melt-in-your mouth brownies, you can eat them while they are still warm; if you like firm, cakelike brownies, let them cool completely in the refrigerator.

Dust with cocoa powder, if desired, and cut into squares.

TIP: Hot chocolate
Be sure to thoroughly cool the melted chocolate; otherwise, it will begin to set the eggs when you add it to the batter.

TIP: Dried apricots
You can also buy semidried apricots. They can be more difficult to find, but I prefer to use the semidried kind because the result is smoother.

MAKES
5 or 6 tartlets

PREPARATION
20 minutes

COOKING TIME
15 minutes

Tomato Tartlets

1 pound (455 g) cherry tomatoes

3 tablespoons coconut sugar (see tip, page 186)

1 sheet (8 ounces/ 230 g) puff pastry

Preheat the oven to 350°F (180°C).

Halve the cherry tomatoes. Put a little olive oil and the tomatoes in a skillet. Sauté them over medium heat for about 2 minutes until the tomatoes soften and skins just begin to wrinkle. Don't cook them too long, or you will have tomato sauce.

Put the coconut sugar in a small saucepan and place it over medium heat. Do not stir. When the sugar begins to caramelize, add the tomatoes and stir gently.

Divide the tomatoes among small ovenproof ramekins. Cut rounds of puff pastry to fit the top of the ramekins and place them on top. Set the ramekins on a rimmed baking sheet. Bake for 15 minutes until the pastry is completely dry and well done.

Remove the tartlets from the oven. Let them cool for a few minutes, then invert them onto individual plates.

Inspiration for these tartlets came from the famous apple dessert tarte Tatin. Half-lunch, half-dessert . . . a true delight!

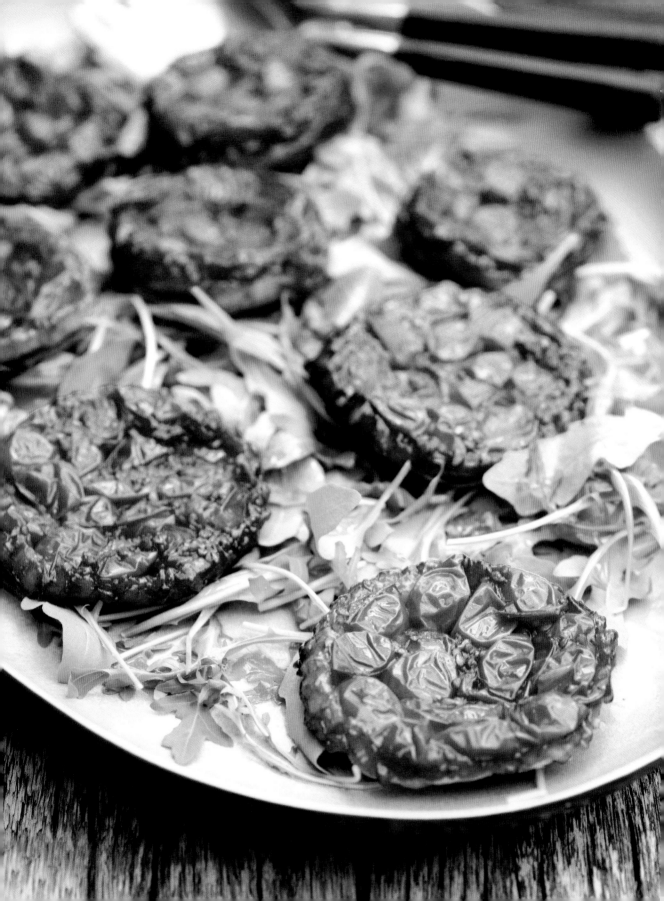

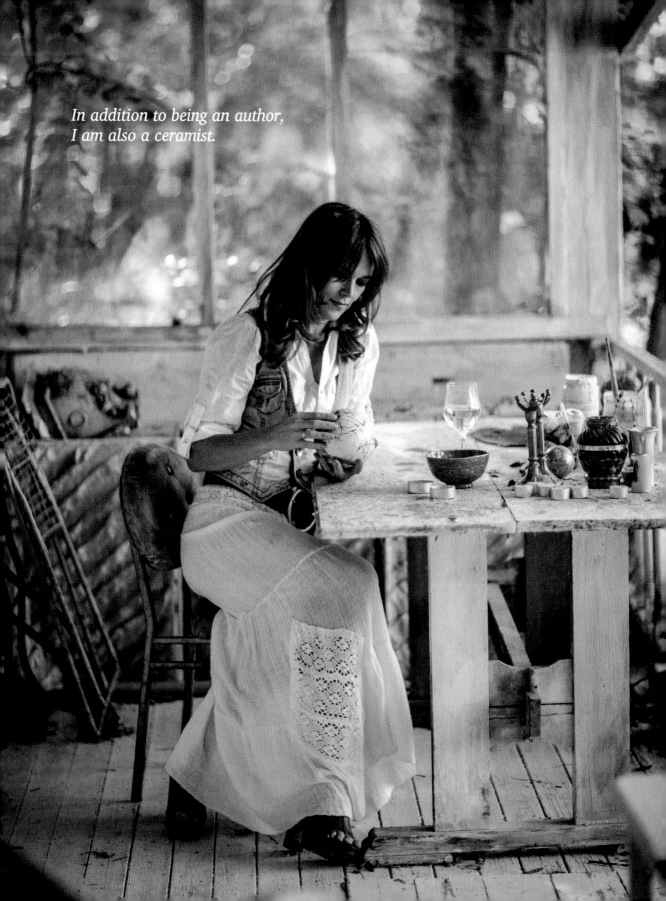

In addition to being an author,
I am also a ceramist.

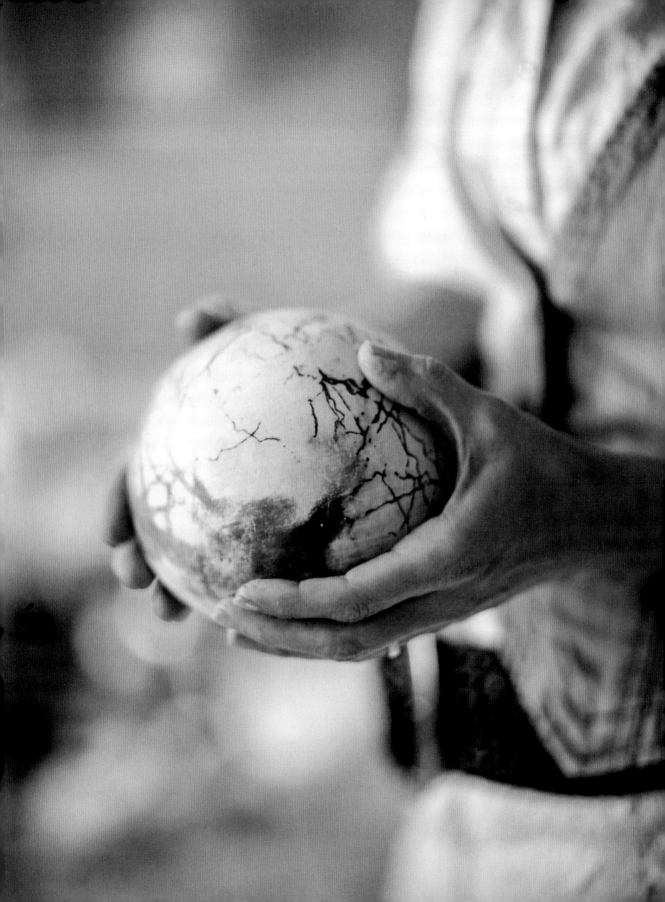

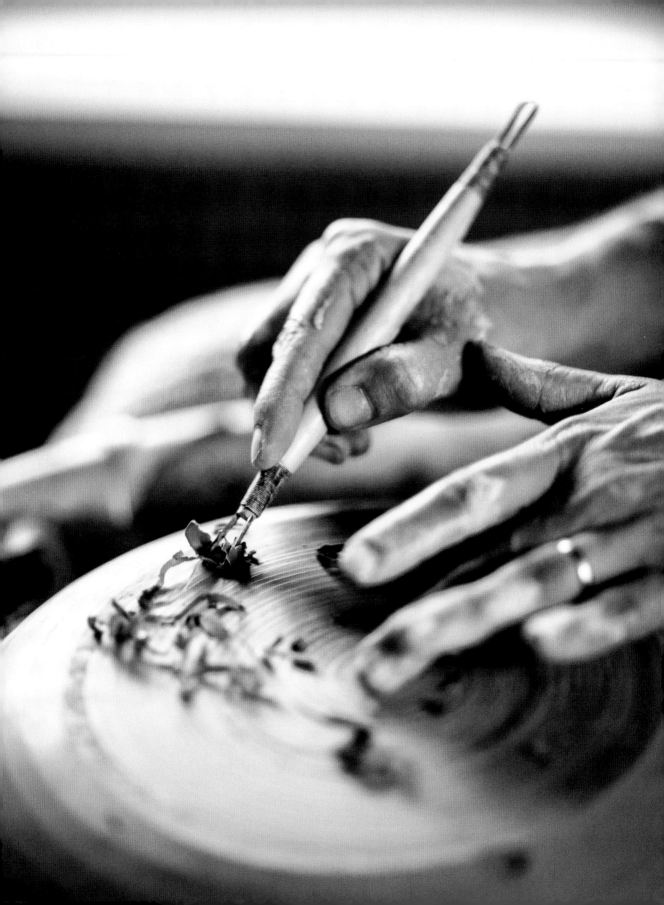

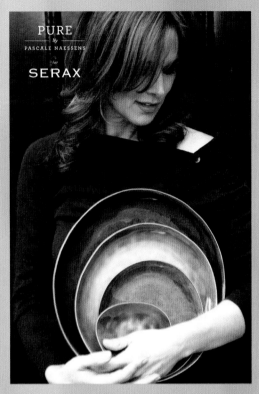

For me, being a ceramist is a logical extension of everything I'm doing—cooking and serving food in a beautiful way to my loved ones.

It is a fantastic challenge, molding that lump of clay on the wheel with your own hands. It requires strength, knowledge, experience, and creativity. This passion led to the development and production of my own professional line, Pure by Pascale Naessens for Serax, which has become an international success. Chefs at celebrated restaurants and home cooks serve food on plates designed by me. I am so thrilled about that.

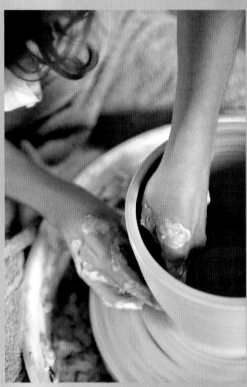

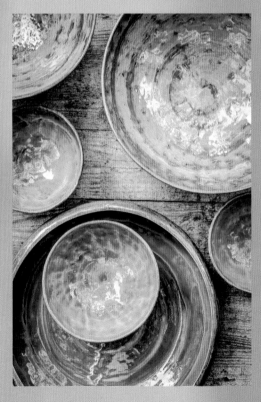

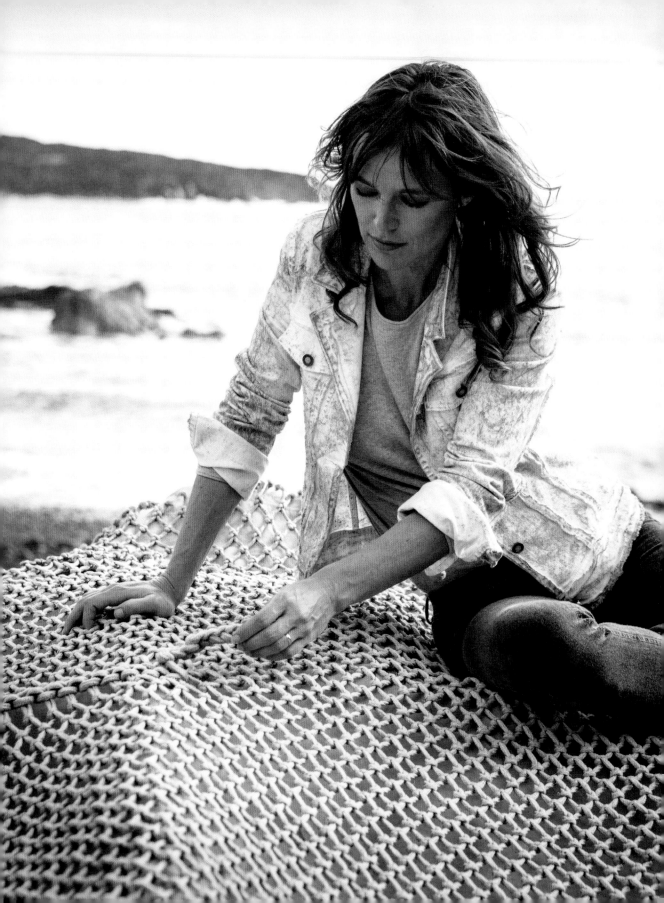

Starting Your Journey

Caminante, no hay camino, se hace camino al andar.
(Stroller, there is no path. Your walk creates the path.)
—ANTONIO MACHADO

A while ago, when I began to learn Spanish, I discovered the verse above. I have thought about it and what Antonio Machado so beautifully expresses: It is exactly what I also think and feel. Don't agonize over what you want to do later, what you want to become, or what you want to achieve. Indeed, how could you know? Can you see the future? Instead, ask yourself: What excites me? What am I feeling now? And do not listen only to your mind: Also listen to your instincts. Your mind could very well mislead you: We grew up in societies with high expectations and prejudices, which are all printed in our minds. Your gut does not take these kind of issues into account. Feel for yourself, act on your feelings, and only then think about what you can do with them.

You have to have courage to make the decision to start on your path. Of course, you may be overcome by fear and doubt at times—it's part of the journey. But the next day, you will find courage again and move on. Stay true to yourself, to your nature, and trust your inner compass. Don't set unreasonable goals; act now and follow your own inspiration.

What job, what studies make you happy? What hobby do you love? What workshop would you like to attend? Nobody will do your work for you. You have to do it yourself. So stop thinking and begin acting.

Start small and move step by step. This applies to everything in life. Have a mindful approach to nutrition, health, beauty, and happiness. Eat food that gives you a feeling of satisfaction. Find work that you enjoy, that fulfills you. Seek to learn about things that excite you. Good choices like these make a person happy, stress-resistant, strong, and healthy.

I personally never set goals; I had no idea what I wanted to do in life, but I had confidence that it would be okay. I never imagined that I would have the life I have today: living with a fantastic man, writing books, cooking, creating my own ceramic line, designing furniture, and more. I don't believe in "predestined" talent. Talent should be cultivated, developed. The path brought me here. And if I can do it, everybody can. You just have to start your journey.

Index of Recipes

Index of Ingredients

www.purepascale.com
We love to hear about your experiences with this way of eating. Visit the website above and contact us via our contact page. Visit our testimonials page for more stories. We're stronger together.

ACKNOWLEDGMENTS

I would like to thank the people and companies who contributed to this book. Without them, I could not have completed this project:

Danielle Westerweel of the Krijn Verwijs company in Yerseke who introduced me to enthusiastic fishermen, people who love their work and products; Jan Kruijsse, who told me everything about seaweed; and Jan Poleij, a professional picker of sea aster and salicornia who took us to one of his secret sandbanks full of these delicious sea plants.

Originally published in Dutch by Lannoo Publishers as *Puur eten 2 dat je gelukkig maakt*

Belgian Edition
Recipes, Texts, Styling, and Concept Layout: Pascale Naessens
Photographers: Roos Mestdagh, Diego Franssens, Wout Hendrickx, Ludo Goossens, and Ramon de Llano
Designer: Katrien Van De Steene—Whitespray bvba
Translator: Marguerite Storms

Abrams Edition
Editor: Laura Dozier
Designer: Danielle Young
Production Manager: True Sims and Anet Sirna-Bruder

Library of Congress Control Number: 2016949535

ISBN: 978-1-4197-2617-0

Printed and bound in the United States
10 9 8 7 6 5 4 3 2 1

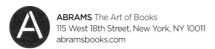

ABRAMS The Art of Books
115 West 18th Street, New York, NY 10011
abramsbooks.com